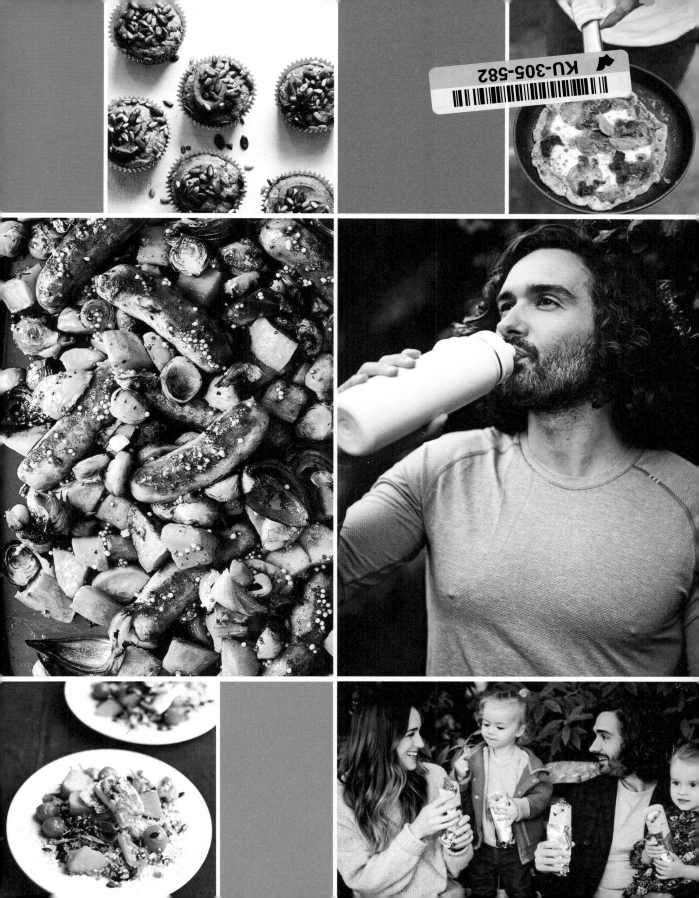

JOE WICKS

FEEL GOOD *Food*

JOE WICKS

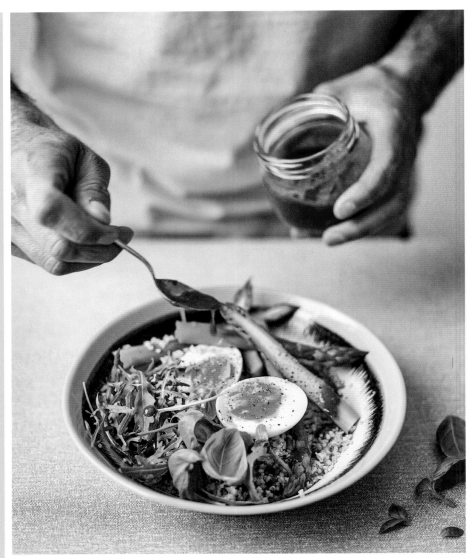

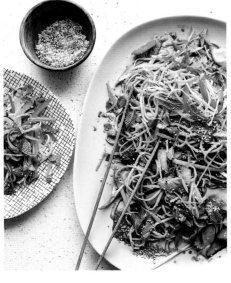

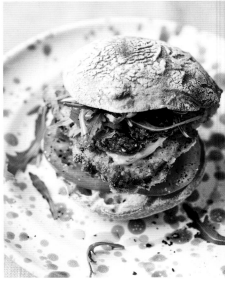

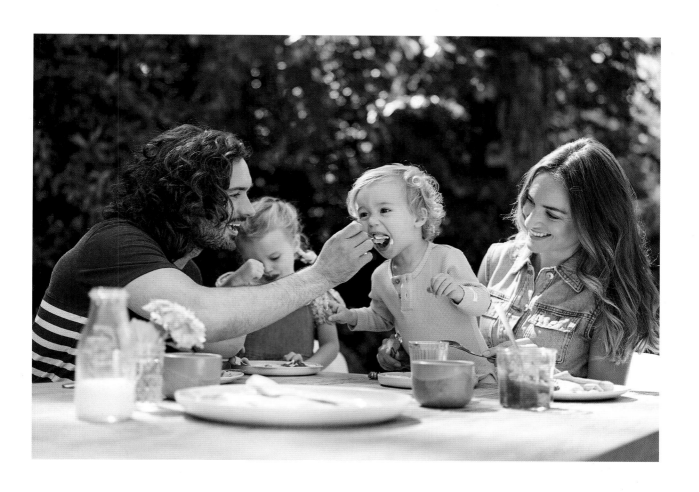

FEEL
GOOD
Food

OVER 100 HEALTHY FAMILY RECIPES

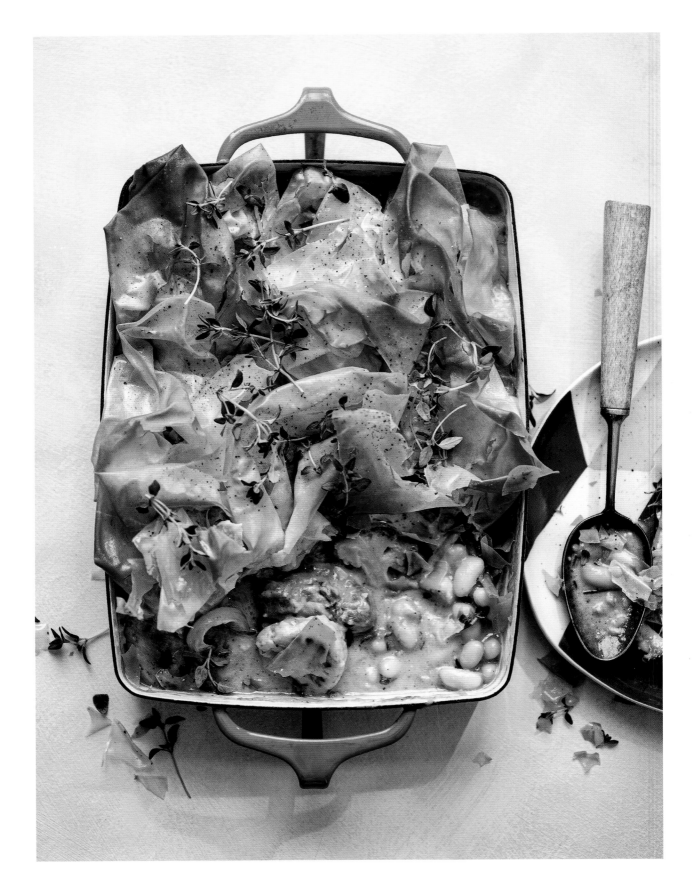

CONTENTS

INTRODUCTION

Welcome to *Feel Good Food*. I'm so excited to share a new collection of incredible recipes to get you and your family feeling energised and happy. Food really does have the power to change our mood for the better. I believe this is more important now than ever.

It's often overlooked just how much the food we eat changes the way we feel on the inside and how this affects our mental health. Good food makes us feel fantastic. It nourishes and energises us and unlocks more potential in us every day. When you really commit to a healthy diet, it can transform your life in so many ways beyond just the physical changes you will see on the outside.

Putting good food in your body every day will increase your energy levels, improve your focus and productivity, help you feel calmer and less stressed, improve your gut health and help you sleep better. Just imagine if you had all of those things in your life today. It would not only improve your confidence and benefit your mental health immensely, but it would also have a positive impact on so many others around you. When you feel happier, less stressed, more patient and calmer, your relationships with others will improve, so everyone wins.

It makes so much sense, doesn't it, when you read all those wonderful benefits, and it seems so easy? Yet eating healthily and being consistent with food is the one thing people struggle with the most. There are times during the year when I find my motivation dips and I have to work harder to get back on track. One thing I've learned about myself, though, is that my motivation to stay active and eat well has changed. My focus used to be on getting lean, staying in shape and looking good, but now it's all about feeling good. I really am a better and happier person when I'm putting good food in my body.

My philosophy around food and nutrition hasn't changed since I started out as a trainer 10 years ago. I still believe a balanced and flexible approach to eating is the most sustainable and enjoyable way of living. By keeping things simple and easy in the kitchen you are able to enjoy the foods you love without restricting yourself.

The key to long term success is simply learning to enjoy cooking. When you enjoy the process of getting in the kitchen and preparing delicious home-cooked food, you soon realise that you don't have to rely on takeaways, ultra-processed foods or

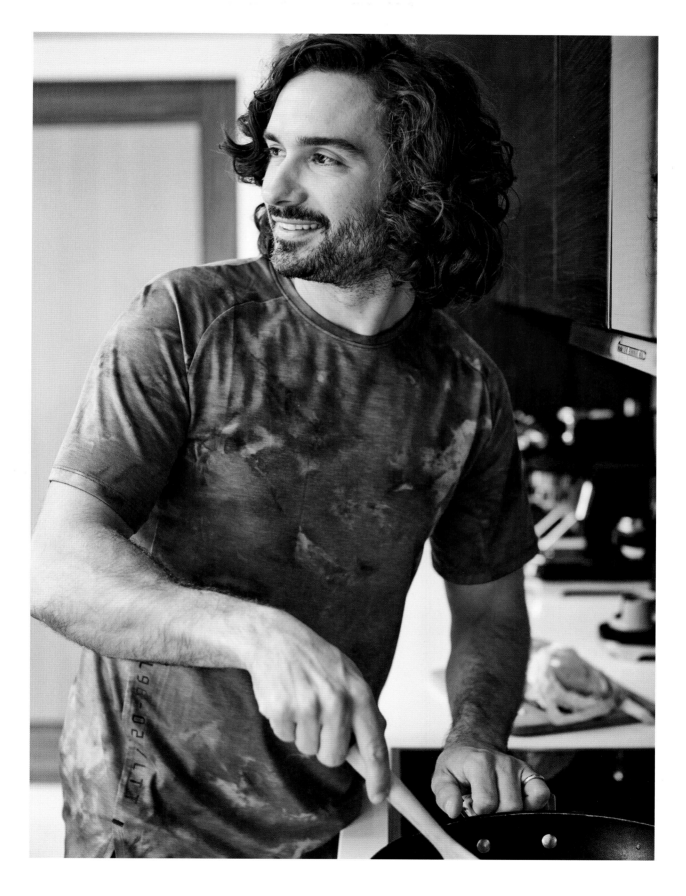

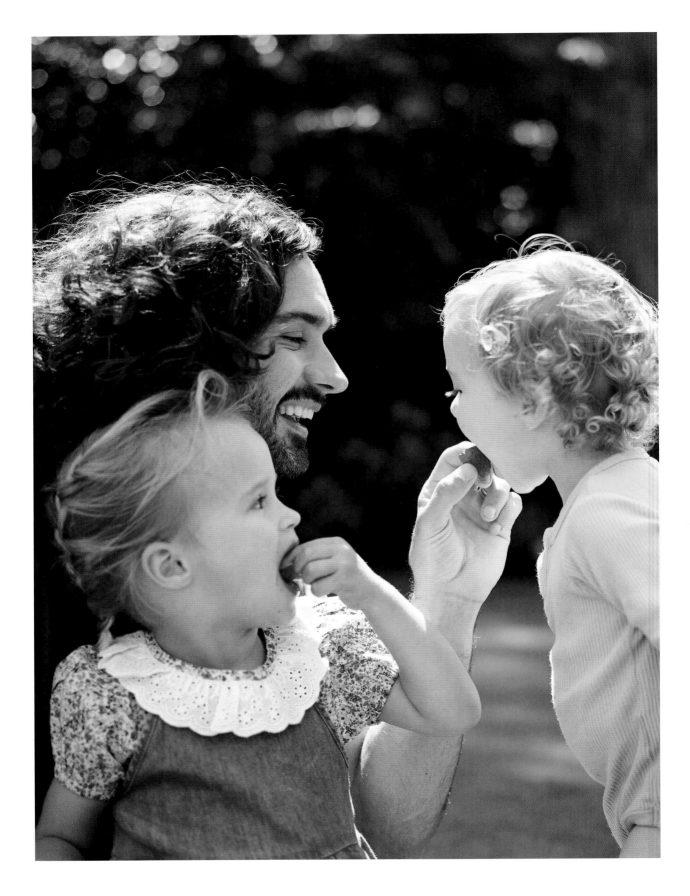

ready meals on the go. As you learn new recipes and styles of cooking, you start to feel empowered and look forward to getting in the kitchen. It's a wonderful feeling to be in control of the food you eat, knowing exactly what it's made from, and it allows you to gain a much better understanding of your body and what it needs to feel energised.

Home cooking, and specifically batch cooking, also leads to a really positive side effect: you are setting yourself up for success. When you make a big portion of curry or chilli, for example, you can store the rest in the fridge and eat it the next day. This is such a simple strategy once you get into the swing of it and is really transformative. It takes some of the stress out of cooking the following day and means you know you've got a healthy meal ready to go the moment you arrive at work or return home. This habit can really help you stay on track with your health and fitness goals.

In *Feel Good Food* I want to bring a bit of joy back into eating and home cooking. I've created these recipes with ingredients that improve your mood and energy levels and help you get healthy for the long term.

I've made the recipes simple and quick, which I think is the most important factor when trying to live well. They also won't stretch your budget or require top-notch kitchen skills, meaning you can get healthy food on the table fast, whether you are cooking for one or for a whole family.

The recipes are tasty and packed with flavour, but are also full of awesome nutrition. With largely inexpensive ingredients, basic cooking techniques, simple steps and minimal washing-up, my recipes will make your life in the kitchen easier.

I hope to show that eating to feel good is not just about eating the things that are good for your body (although that definitely helps!), it's about learning to enjoy the process and appreciate both the food you eat and the fact that you've made it yourself. In these new recipes, I've tried to combine the most nutritious ingredients in exciting and inventive ways so you get maximum flavour and maximum enjoyment out of them. You can feel good on the inside and happy on the outside, too!

Here's to feeling good with *Feel Good Food*. Thanks again for trying my new recipes. I hope you love them all and enjoy the journey to a healthy, happy mind and body.

Love,

Joe

KICK-START YOUR POSITIVITY: JOE'S BUILDING BLOCKS FOR FEEL GOOD EATING

REDUCE MEAT INTAKE

Focus on choosing lean meats, fish and eggs for their mood-enhancing nutrients.

EAT MORE PLANTS

Fresh fruit and veggies should be the backbone of your diet.

EAT MORE WHOLE-GRAINS

Wholegrains are best for keeping your mood and sleep patterns stable.

PREP LIKE A BOSS

Cooking from scratch for yourself and your family can make you feel good and get you healthier, too.

CHOOSE 'SLOW-RELEASE' CARBOHYDRATES

Slow, complex carbs, such as oats, brown rice, beans, apples or carrots, are a steady source of brain fuel.

MINIMISE ULTRA-PROCESSED FOODS

Avoid fizzy, sugary drinks, instant noodles, crisps, and store-bought biscuits (and at the same time avoid trans fats, too).

DON'T FORGET DAIRY

Consumed in the right amounts, dairy products provide essential proteins.

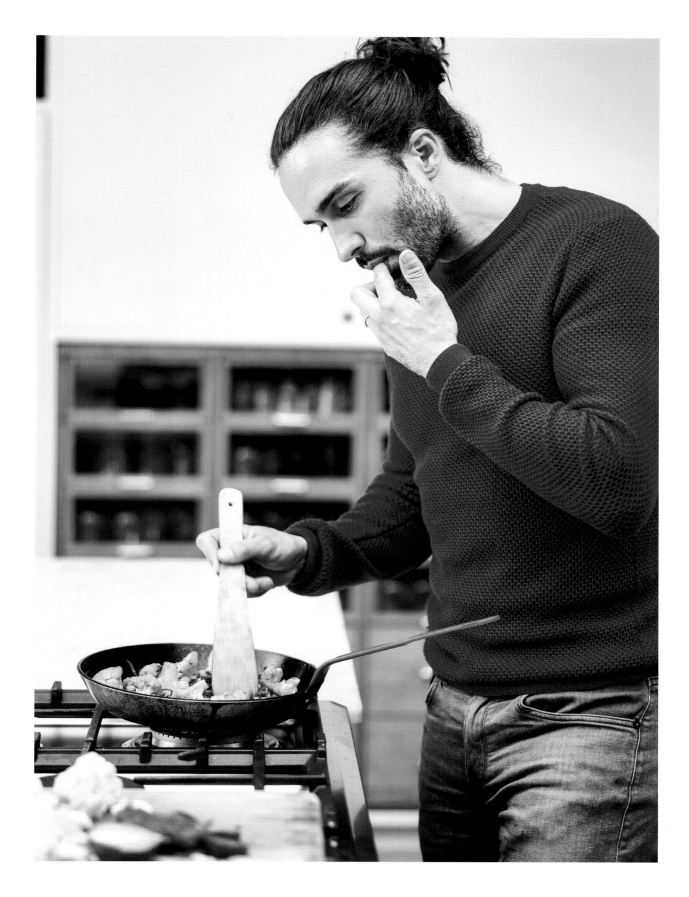

THE LINK BETWEEN FOOD AND MOOD

Do you notice a positive shift in your mood when you have a day of healthy eating? Have you ever wondered why it makes you feel good – not just physically, but mentally? Feeling more energised is obvious because we know that the food we consume is fuel for our bodies, but did you know about the link between the gut and the brain?

When you hear the word 'serotonin' you might initially think of the feel good chemical that is released in the brain after physical activity. You may be surprised to learn that that 90% of serotonin is actually produced in the gut. I couldn't believe this myself and only found it out very recently. Knowing this, it's easy now to see just how much the food we eat can affect our mood and mental health, both positively and negatively based on the choices we make.

In my personal experience, whenever I have a proper blow-out and just eat everything in sight, I feel the physical effects almost immediately. Things like fizzy drinks, tubs of ice cream and deep-fried foods probably do me in the most. I usually become super-bloated, with uncomfortable trapped wind, feel really lethargic and sometimes can even get cramps and diarrhoea in the night. I feel absolutely no guilt emotionally when this happens because I love my food and think it's nice to have treats from time to time. However, they serve as a reminder as to why I want to eat better and put good healthy food in my body most of the time. It gets me back into the kitchen the next day to prepare a nutritious meal, that's for sure, and I get back on track.

Aside from the physical impact that sugary, ultra-processed and deep-fried foods have on my body, I also feel what can only be described as a food hangover the next day, where I feel a noticeable shift in my mood. I'm usually feeling really tired even if I've had a good night's sleep, my mood is low and I generally feel flat. I am less patient with people around me and get irritated easily. This is without doubt a result of the direct link between my gut and my brain – affecting my serotonin levels.

Ultimately, no one has a perfect diet 365 days a year, but it's good to know that we have the ability to control the way we feel and give ourselves a chance to boost our mood with good food and exercise. It's very easy to turn to junk food when we feel down, stressed, anxious or depressed, but if we learn to turn to the good stuff instead we can really change our vibe and lift that cloud in our mind. And even if it's only temporary, it's worth a try, right? We deserve to be happy, so let's give our gut a chance to tell our brain we are in a good mood.

Food fuels both body and mind. We eat nutritious foods so that our bodies can grow, repair and function well, but our brain needs nutritious foods too, accounting for about 20% of our daily energy requirements. When we choose nutritious foods, we're providing our bodies and brains with the building blocks we need to be at our best. From vitamins and minerals to healthy fats and fibre, all nutrients play a role in brain health and function, and therefore impact our mood.

So, what foods should we be eating to support better mental wellbeing? A big part of having a healthy diet is eating a wide variety of different plants. Eating more fruit and vegetables, as well as being extremely good for your body, has been linked to lower rates of depression, so it's good for your mood too.

Here are some known mood-boosting ingredients. Try them out whenever you are feeling in need of a bit of positivity and see how they make you feel good:

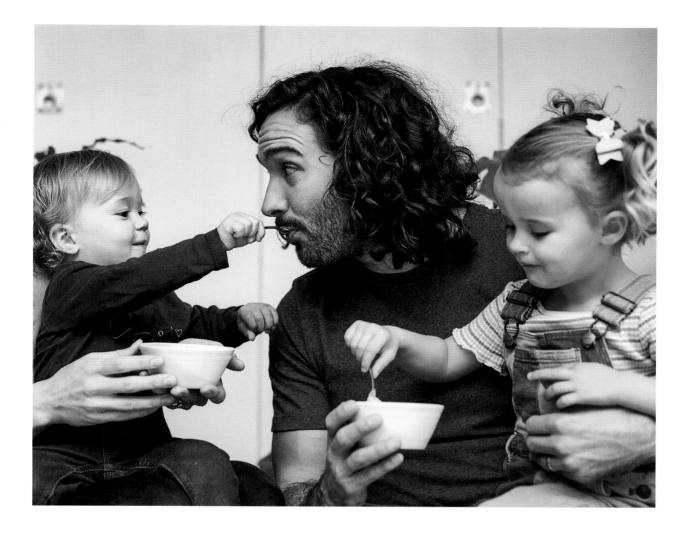

Bananas: These are a great source of natural sugar, prebiotic fibre and vitamin B6, which work to keep your blood sugars and mood stable. Low blood sugar can lead to mood swings and irritability. So, a banana a day can really make you feel good.

Oats: Another stabiliser of your blood sugars and an excellent way to start a day, the fibre in oats can help stabilise your mood and keep you full up and less likely to snack. They are also full of iron, which has been shown to turn around fatigue, sluggishness and low mood.

Dark chocolate: This is rich in compounds that increase the feel good chemicals in your brain. It's also sugary, so while you do get a mood-boosting hit from it, limit it to a few small squares at a time.

WHY WE CHOOSE HEALTHY OPTIONS

Choosing heathier options doesn't mean sacrificing flavour or enjoyment. Instead, it means choosing the things that will make you feel better and more energised in the long run. The more consistent you are with healthy choices, the easier it becomes – you'll get into good habits. Eventually, it becomes a lifestyle you love living.

INTRODUCTION

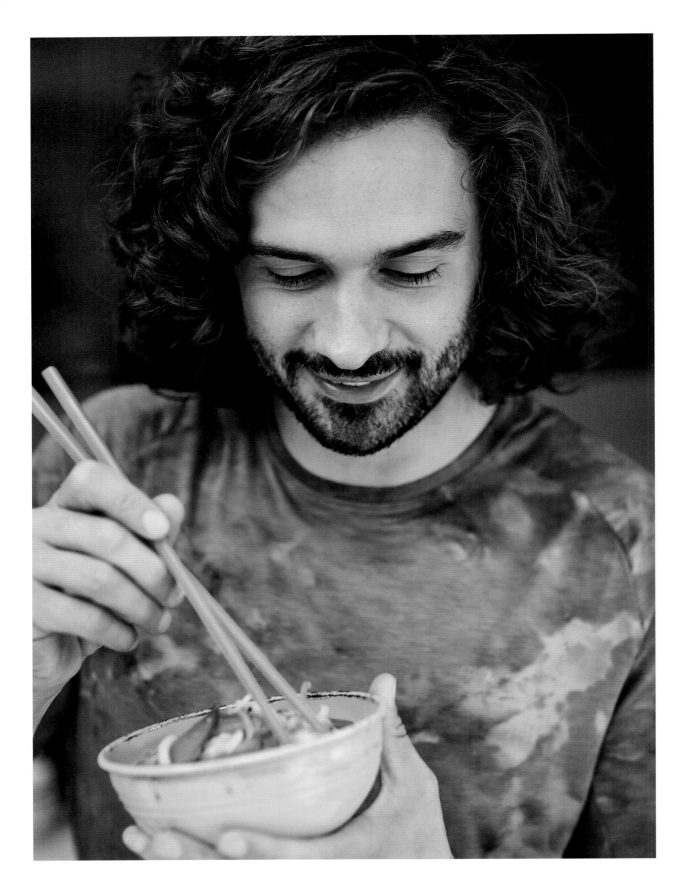

Berries: Fresh berries, particularly blueberries, are rich in antioxidants and other disease-fighting compounds which can reduce the risk of depression and inflammation, and help combat oxidative stress in your body.

Nuts and seeds: As well as being high in plant-based proteins, healthy fats and fibre, they also provide tryptophan, which is an amino acid responsible for producing serotonin – the mood-boosting chemical. Good sources are almonds, walnuts, cashews, peanuts, pumpkin seeds, sesame seeds and sunflower seeds.

Beans and lentils: Full of feel good nutrients, as well as being excellent sources of plant-based protein and fibre, pulses are superfoods. They are full of B vitamins, which are key mood-boosting nutrients, as well as being good sources of zinc, magnesium and selenium, which are also known to elevate your spirits.

Fatty fish (such as salmon and tuna): These are full of omega-3 fatty acids, which are essential for brain development, but are now known to be linked to reducing the risk of depression. Try to eat at least 100g a few times a week.

Fermented foods (such as yoghurt, kimchi, sauerkraut or miso): It has been suggested that the probiotics in fermented foods can also boost mood while improving your gut health, since serotonin is largely produced in your gut. Research is beginning to show a link between healthy gut bacteria and lower rates of depression.

Eggs: Eggs are a fantastic source of nutrients that are linked to improved brain health, including vitamins B6, B12, folate and choline. Choline is particuarly important for our bodies to regulate mood and memory.

Oranges: Foods that are high in vitamin C can help defend your brain against the damaging effect of free radicals – which can cause oxidative stress – and improve focus and decision speed. You can get almost all the vitamin C you need in a day from eating just one orange. Other foods rich in vitamin C are bell peppers, strawberries and tomatoes.

ON COMFORT FOOD

With this book, I wanted to find options that made me feel like I was treating myself, but that didn't make me feel lacking in energy afterwards. A treat should be just that – a comforting lift for your mind that's also good for your body!

I have included a chapter on how to make healthier versions of common takeaways. Foods that we often crave or those that we grab when we're out and about or in a hurry: tacos, burgers, pizzas, even pre-packaged 'health' snacks, such as salted or flavoured nuts. These meals and snacks can easily be prepared at home for a fraction of the cost and a fraction of the calories, and with many more health-beneficial ingredients included. With my versions, you lose none of the pleasure or comfort and none of the flavour, but you satisfy that craving with something that's good for you too.

ON FAMILY FOOD

Nothing makes me happier than seeing Indie and Marley enjoying food and being adventurous with new things. From the very first few months of eating as babies, we were introducing them to new herbs, spices and textures. This has led them to be really brave when it comes to trying new recipes and flavours. We love sitting and enjoying food together, so we aim to eat the same meals at the same time. We rarely make a separate meal for them and I think this is really important when it comes to children's nutrition and avoiding fussy eating in kids. I'm really passionate about sharing this message because, as parents, we are their biggest role models and they constantly learn and take inspiration from us.

I believe the most effective way of encouraging healthy eating is by getting children involved in the cooking and having some fun with it. My kids won't go near boiled or steamed veg, but when I let them sprinkle some Cajun spice or paprika on their broccoli and cauliflower and roast it in the oven they absolutely love the stuff. If you can engage your little ones in food from a young age, you are setting them up for a healthy future, too.

To help with this, I have created some really simple and fun child-friendly recipes to get you going. It can be a messy business, but just see it as fun activity and a chance to connect with them. Even the simplest of things, such as letting your kids stir the porridge or add berries on top, can sometimes be enough to light up their little faces. Indie and Marley have helped me make pasta, muffins, mini pizzas and pancakes and there's no doubt that it's got them super interested in food.

Why not try letting your kids top their favourite pizza, build their own breakfast bowl or throw together their own taco ingredients? Including a wide range of foods, colours, flavours and textures in their meals means that they'll feel interested and excited about what they're eating. Food really does become an adventure and you are also giving them skills which could change their lives.

> The most effective way of encouraging healthy eating is by getting children involved in the cooking and having some fun with it.

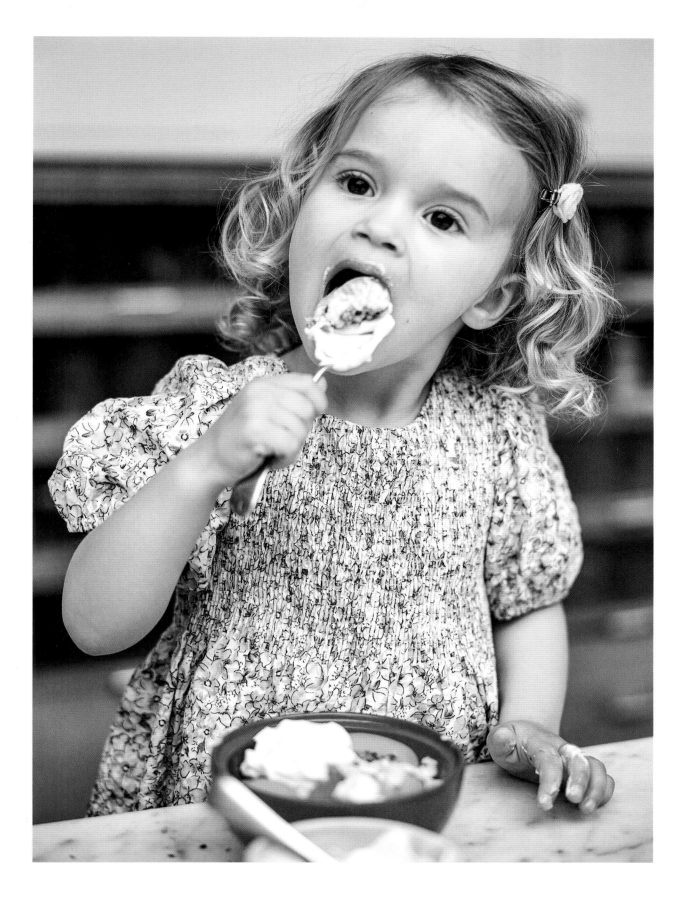

JOE'S TIPS FOR FEEL GOOD LIVING

RELAXATION

Don't forget about time out – try some mindfulness and meditation.

SIT DOWN TO EAT

Take your time over it – have mealtimes with the family if you can.

MAKE TIME TO MOVE

15–30 minutes of activity every day.

DRINK MORE WATER

Don't forget this one – especially when exercising!

STRETCH

Staying supple and mobile helps with everyday aches and pains.

EAT REGULARLY

3 meals a day plus healthy snack choices.

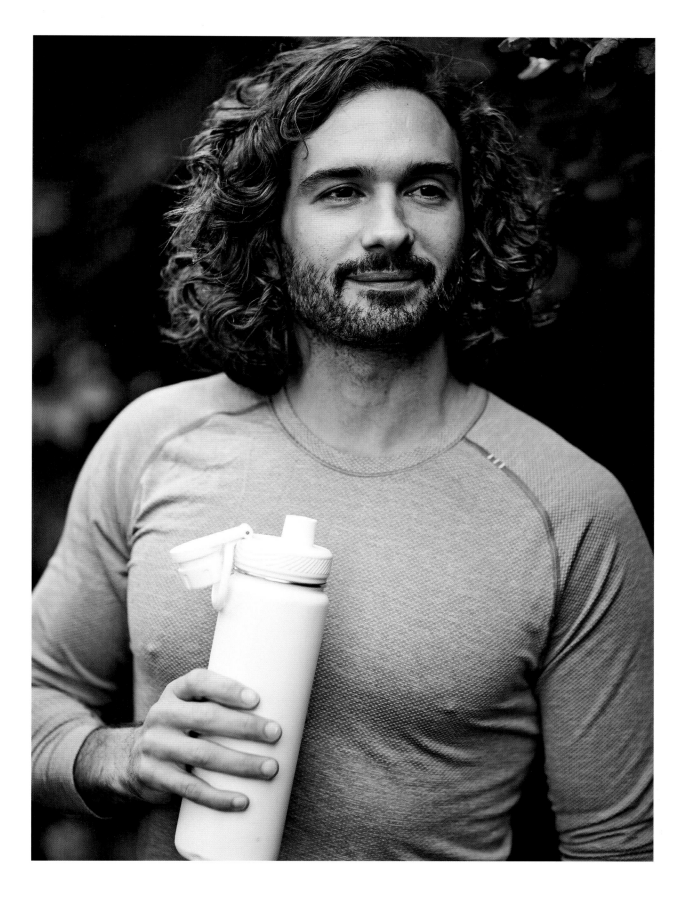

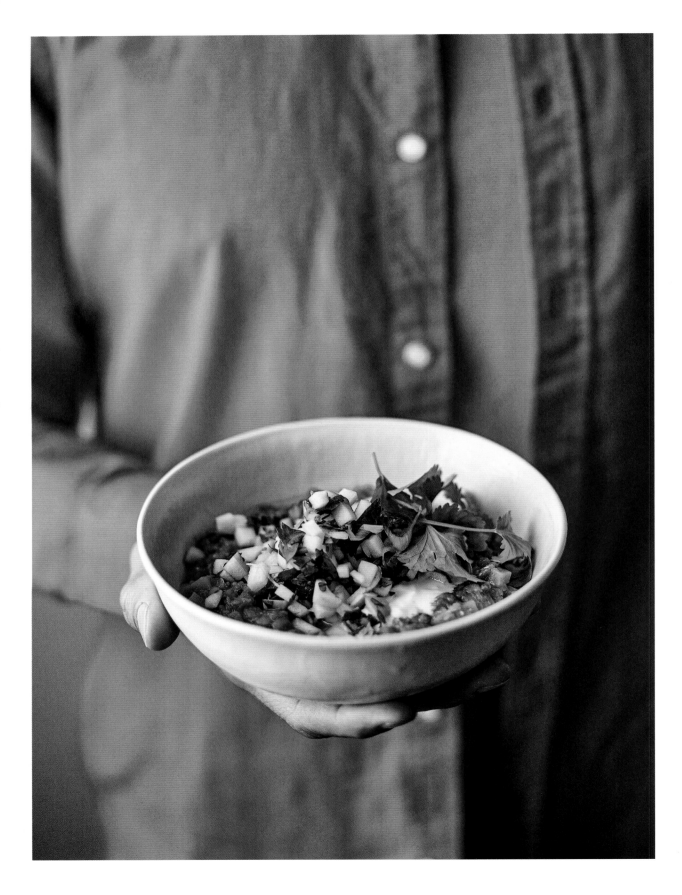

THE BUILDING BLOCKS OF A HEALTHY DIET

Understanding what the essential building blocks for our diets are, and why they work together to help you feel good and give you energy, is key to learning to eat well.

There are six main classes of nutrients that the body needs. These are: proteins, carbohydrates, fats, fibre, micronutrients (vitamins and minerals) and water. It is important that you consume all these nutrients on a daily basis to help build your body and maintain your health.

1 PROTEINS

These are needed in our diets for growth (they are especially important for children, growing teens and pregnant women) and to improve our immune system function. They also play an important role in making essential hormones and enzymes, in tissue repair, preserving lean muscle mass, and supplying energy in those times when carbohydrates are not available.

The main sources of protein are meat, chicken, eggs, beans and lentils, nuts, fish and dairy.

There is more protein in animal sources than in plant-based sources, but even though plant proteins are considered incomplete, you can combine several sources, such as pulses, legumes and grains, to get all of your essential amino acids in one meal.

2 FIBRE

Fibre is actually a mixture of different carbohydrates that are not digested like other nutrients but pass through the gut nearly unchanged. It makes our food bulky, filling us up and helping it to pass through the gut, and slows the absorption of nutrients into the bloodstream.

Foods rich in fibre include wholegrains (wheat flour, bulgur wheat, oats), vegetables such as cabbage or carrots, fruits such as bananas or avocados, and peas and beans.

3 CARBOHYDRATES

Carbs are an amazing source of energy for the body. Up to 65% of our energy comes from carbohydrates. For the brain, kidneys, central nervous system and muscles to function properly, they all need carbohydrates, so don't be scared of them.

Some of the main sources of carbohydrate are bread, wheat, potatoes of all kinds, rice, pasta, banana, sugar, sweet fruits and honey. Other foods, such as vegetables, beans, nuts and seeds, do contain carbohydrates, but in lesser amounts.

Carbs are sometimes given a bad reputation. However, it's important to remember that not all carbs are bad. We need them to function. Our brain needs the glucose that comes from starchy carbs. Without it, we can be very fatigued and lack concentration and focus.

When it comes to quality carbohydrates, there are some good choices you can make: Choose natural sources of sugar over refined sugars; choose brown rice over white rice; choose higher-fibre wholemeal or buckwheat pasta over white pasta; or choose sourdough bread over processed bread (or make your own – if you use wholegrain flour and throw in a few seeds, the loaf will be rich in fibre and vitamin E, too). And remember, you can really pack a sandwich with lots of delicious, healthy ingredients to complement the carbs, so enjoy them.

4 FATS

Fats are often given a bad rap in the dieting world, but they really shouldn't be. Fat plays an important role in the human body and some fatty acids, such as omega-3 found in oily fish and flax seed, are considered essential because they cannot be made in the body and must come from our diet. Fat is also a fantastic source of energy, which can help regulate blood sugar levels. Try to eat it in moderation alongside protein and carbohydrates.

Fat is found in meat, chicken, dairy products, avocado, cooking oils and fats, fish and nuts. It's important to get a good variety of fat in your diet, so don't overthink it too much and just try to eat some of the above foods during your day.

5 MICRO NUTRIENTS

Vitamins

Vitamins are present in small amounts in foods and are necessary for the body to function effectively – they are sometimes called 'protective foods'. They are grouped together because they are a vital factor in our diets.

Vitamins are classified into two groups:

Fat-soluble vitamins (A, D, E and K) are soluble in fats and fat solvents. They are not soluble in water. So these are utilised only if there is enough fat in the body.

Water-soluble vitamins (B, C and folic acid) are soluble in water and so they cannot be stored in the body.

Minerals

We need minerals to ensure the health and correct working of our soft tissues, fluids and bones. Minerals include calcium, iron, iodine, fluorine, phosphorus, potassium, zinc, selenium and sodium.

The best sources of micronutrients in our diets are fruits and vegetables. These two food groups contain essential vitamins and minerals. Animal sources are also good sources of micronutrients, but an adequate micronutrient intake can only be achieved through a balanced diet that includes plenty of fruits and vegetables.

6 WATER

Don't forget to drink lots of water! Water is essential for life and everything in the body works better when it's properly hydrated. We can live without solid food for a few weeks, but we cannot live without water for more than a few days. An adult needs about 2–3 litres of water every day. My top tip is to always carry a metal refillable bottle that you can top up a few times throughout the day.

THE PERFECT DIET

The truth is, there is no one perfect one-size-fits-all diet for everybody. What might work for someone else may not work as well for you. The most important thing to do is to eat to feel energised. You may feel better eating a lower carb diet and getting more energy from fats and protein. The best thing is to try things out and see how your body reacts and feels. If certain food groups make you feel sluggish, bloated or unhappy, then just reduce them in your diet. You'll soon work out what foods make you feel good and then you'll be cruising along.

FORWARD PLANNING

Keep your kitchen stocked so that eating well becomes easier. If your kitchen cupboard, fridge or freezer always contains the right foods, you're less likely to turn to the wrong foods. I try to keep most of the following items in stock at all times.

Cupboard

almonds (flaked or skin-on)

apple cider vinegar or
red wine vinegar

artichokes in oil

baking powder

black pepper

breadcrumbs (panko)

bulgur wheat

coconut milk

couscous

dark chocolate

dried noodles

eggs

flour (plain wholemeal)

honey

oils (light and extra-virgin olive oil,
vegetable oil, sesame oil)

packets of pre-cooked brown rice

ketchup/tomato sauce/passata

pasta (different types)

peanuts

pine nuts

porridge oats

rice (long grain and risotto)

sea salt

seeds (pumpkin, sesame)

dried herbs and spices (chilli flakes,
paprika, cumin and coriander,
cinnamon, dried oregano)

stock cubes

soy sauce

sun-dried tomatoes in oil

tahini

tins or pouches of cooked pulses
(cannellini beans, lentils, chickpeas,
black beans, kidney beans)

tinned tomatoes/sweetcorn

walnuts

Freezer

berries (all kinds: blueberries,
strawberries, raspberries)

broad beans

chopped mango

chopped red peppers

peas

chopped spinach

sweetcorn

good-quality vegetarian or meat
sausages

wholemeal flatbreads

Fridge

butter or coconut oil

filo pastry

chipotle or harissa paste

crème fraîche

feta cheese

fish (small amounts, as and when
needed)

gnocchi

halloumi

hot sauce

meat (small amounts, as and when
needed)

milk (of choice)

miso paste

mozzarella

mustard

nut butters

olives

paneer

Parmesan cheese

roasted peppers

ricotta

Thai curry pastes

tofu

tomato purée concentrate

natural yoghurt

Fresh

aubergines

bananas

beetroot

bread (wholemeal/wholegrain)

broccoli

butternut squash

carrots

cauliflower

chillies

courgettes

cucumber

garlic

ginger

herbs (basil, coriander, mint, parsley,
dill, thyme)

kale

leeks

lemons, limes and oranges

lettuce

mushrooms

onions (red and brown)

peaches

peppers

potatoes (white and sweet)

root vegetables (carrots, parsnips)

spring onions

tomatoes

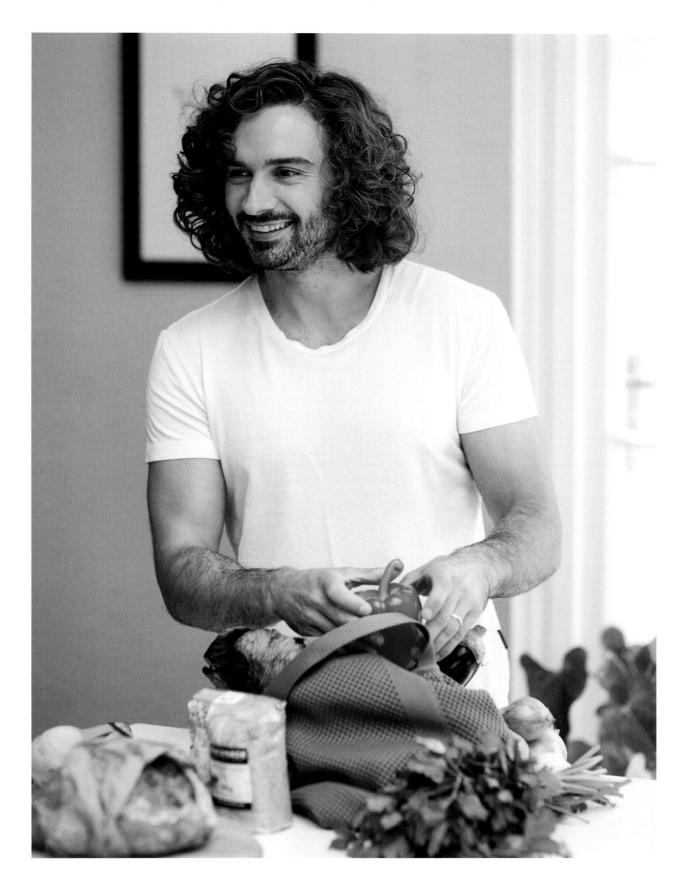

USEFUL INGREDIENTS FOR A FEEL GOOD DIET

These are the foods you will find a lot of in this book – they form the basis of the recipes I have chosen for you. They are all packed with nutrients and will help you feel good and stay healthy. Not everyone is into the science behind why these ingredients are heroes, but, for those who are, here's an explanation…

Apples

Apples are high in pectin, a type of soluble fibre that may help to reduce cholesterol levels, and also contain insoluble fibre – both help feed your beneficial gut bacteria. By keeping the peel on apples, we keep the part of the fruit that contains the highest level of antioxidants, such as quercetin, which has been linked to improved heart health.

Artichokes

Artichokes contain a high level of inulin – a prebiotic which can help feed the good bacteria in your digestive system, promoting gut health and boosting the feel good chemicals in the brain.

Asparagus

Asparagus is rich in vitamin K and a source of folic acid. It can also act as a prebiotic, meaning it feeds the beneficial gut bacteria, which, in turn, has a positive effect on mood.

Aubergines

This is a good source of fibre and also manganese (which helps form and maintain healthy bones) and rich in polyphenols (antioxidants, which may reduce inflammation).

Avocados

Avocado is a great source of monounsaturated fats (which may support heart health), vitamin E (which helps maintain healthy skin and supports the immune system, absorbs free radicals and keeps red blood cells healthy), and fibre (which aids digestion, supports gut health and helps with control of blood sugars).

Bananas

Bananas contain plenty of fibre and potassium. Potassium helps muscles contract, supports nervous system function, aids digestion, and regulates blood pressure and bodily pH. They are proven mood boosters, too, and will certainly help turn a frown upside down.

Beetroot

Beetroot contains nitrates, which are converted to nitrogen oxide in the body, a compound which helps dilate blood vessels and may lead to reduced blood pressure. This can also improve exercise endurance by improving the flow of oxygen in the bloodstream to the muscles.

Berries (particularly blueberries)

Blueberries are high in anthocyanins (compounds that may have anti-inflammatory properties) which may be the reason why they have been found to improve heart health in scientific studies. If you can't find them fresh, buy them frozen. When frozen at their peak ripeness they retain the maximum amount of mood-boosting and disease-fighting antioxidants.

Black beans

High in fibre and protein, black beans keep you feeling full for longer. They're also a great source of folate, which is vital for our brains and nervous systems.

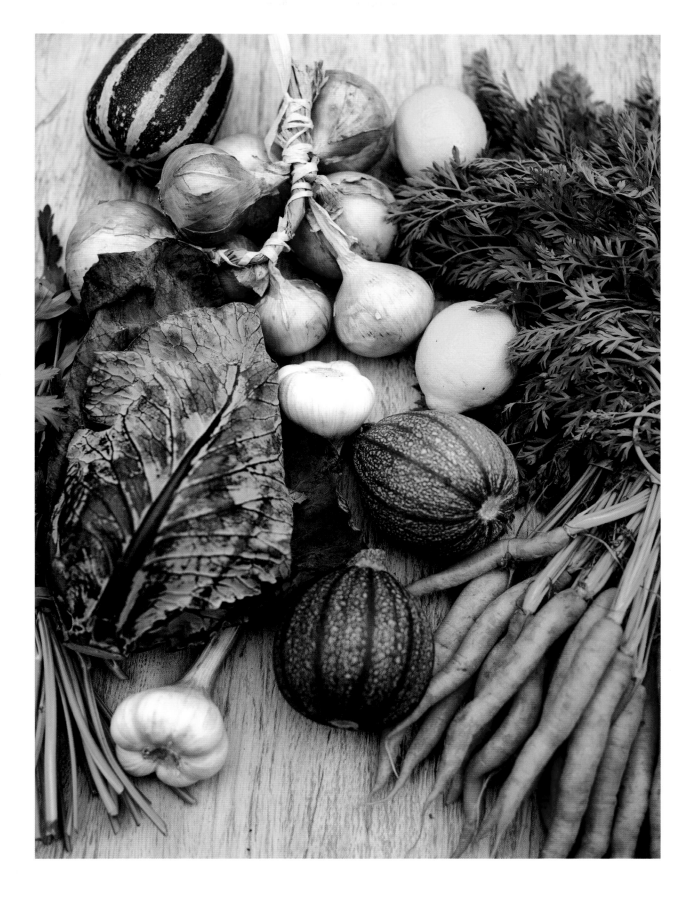

Broccoli

Broccoli has more protein than most veg and is high in vitamins C and K.

Bulgur wheat

A wholegrain, bulgur wheat is quite quick to cook and a good source of fibre, which promotes fullness and better gut and digestive health.

Butternut squash

Butternut squash, as well as being a good source of fibre, contains carotenoids (a type of antioxidant), which are converted to vitamin A in the body (used for eye and skin health and improved immune function).

Carrots

Carrots contain betacarotene, a carotenoid that is used to make vitamin A by our bodies. This, along with lutein, can help maintain eye health. Eating carrots with a source of fat (oil or yoghurt, for instance) helps the body absorb the vitamin A they contain.

Cheese

Choose lower-fat options, such as creamy ricotta, which is high in protein and a good source of calcium, as these are great for bone health and muscle function. It's also a good idea to choose strongly flavoured cheeses, such as feta, so that you only need a small amount to deliver that satisfying cheesy taste.

Cherries

Cherries contain anthocyanins that give them their red colour – these are antioxidants, which may help reduce inflammation.

Chia seeds

Chia seeds contain soluble fibre (that's the reason they swell and thicken when mixed with liquid), which is great for your digestive health. They are also a plant-based source of omega-3 fatty acids, which are important for heart and brain health.

Chickpeas

Chickpeas are an amazing low-fat, plant-based source of protein, which are also rich in fibre and folate (great for gut health,

general wellbeing, controlling blood sugar, keeping you full, lowering cholesterol, improving brain and nervous system function, cell division and forming healthy red blood cells). What a superfood!

Chocolate

Dark chocolate is satisfying when you've got a sugar craving, but it's also a good source of fibre and protein, rich in iron and high in flavanols, which may be beneficial for heart health. Dark chocolate (eaten in moderation) is good for gut health and for boosting mood.

Cinnamon

This delicious warming spice is thought to have anti-inflammatory and antioxidant properties and some studies have shown that it may help mop up harmful free-radicals that do damage to the cells in your body.

Dates

Full of micronutrients and fibre, dates help slow the absorption of sugar into the bloodstream, avoiding blood sugar spikes.

Haricot beans

These are a low-fat, plant-based source of protein and fibre, and are high in folate (a B-vitamin that is needed for making red and white blood cells and for cell division).

Coconut oil

This tastes great, but should be kept to a minimum. It is useful for vegans, but high in saturated fat and will therefore increase cholesterol in the body. A little a day is completely fine, but you may want to try olive oil, seed and nut butters instead.

Eggs

A cheap and versatile source of protein, riboflavin, vitamin B12 and choline. Good for brain health, mood and memory.

Fish

Fish is a fantastic low-fat source of protein, phosphorous, niacin and vitamin B12, so do try to regularly include some in your diet (at least 2 portions a week, one of which should be oily fish). Oily fish, such as salmon or mackerel, has been proven to be good for low mood – the DHA omega-3 fats it contains are responsible for this.

Ginger

A very versatile spice. Ginger may alleviate the symptoms of a cold (make a ginger tea from the grated fresh root – it encourages perspiration and can therefore be used to treat feverish conditions and it also appears to have antiviral effects). It is also soothing on the stomach and reduces the symptoms associated with motion sickness, including dizziness, nausea and cold sweats. It's also good for upset stomachs and dyspepsia. Ginger has a long reputation as a carminative, a substance that promotes the elimination of excess gas from the digestive system, and is known to sooth the intestinal tract. An anti-inflammatory, it is suggested it may also support heart health as well as helping to manage cholesterol levels, reduce damage to the arteries and lower high blood pressure – all of which benefits the heart and cardiovascular system.

Mango

Mango helps promote healthy digestion and is a good source of vitamins A and C.

Miso

Miso is made from fermented soybeans. It is a probiotic, which means it contains good bacteria that may be beneficial for gut health, and improving mood.

Oats

Oats contain healthy fats, fibre, protein and carbohydrates, which are all necessary for a wholesome balanced breakfast. The fibre content of oats can lead to increased satiety meaning you'll stay fuller for longer. They also contain beta glucan, a type of soluble fibre, which can help lower LDL cholesterol leading to better heart health.

Prawns

Prawns are an excellent low-fat source of protein, and are also rich in vitamins B12 and E.

Soya

Contains all nine of the essential amino acids needed to build lean muscle plus healthy monounstaurated and polyunsaturated fats.

Spinach

Spinach is an all-round good guy – rich in folate (needed for forming healthy red blood cells, and maintaining healthy brain and nervous system function), manganese (to help certain enzymes function in the body, protect our cells from damage from free radicals, and to help form and maintain healthy bones), and vitamins A (eye health, skin health and immune function) and K (for wound healing and bone health).

Tofu and tempeh

Tofu is a low-fat, plant-based source of protein that has been linked to improved heart health (from a reduction in LDL cholesterol) and bone health. Tofu and tempeh are great sources of plant-based iron, calcium, zinc and antioxidants.

Tomatoes (fresh and sun-dried)

Tomatoes are full of lycopene, an antioxidant that may be beneficial for cardiovascular health. Sun-dried tomatoes are a brilliant store-cupboard ingredient to have around. Like little flavour bombs, they are full of vitamin C and will pep up so many meals.

Lamb

Lamb is rich in iron and zinc, which are both key for healthy growth and development. It contains plenty of iron in a form that is more easily accessed by the body than the iron found in plant-based sources, which is key for healthy growth and development. Lamb also contains niacin, which helps the body convert nutrients to energy.

Lentils

Lentils are a great source of prebiotic fibre, which feeds your beneficial gut bacteria to support good gut health.

Olives

Olives are high in vitamin E, which helps maintain healthy skin and supports the immune system. They also contain healthy fats, which may support heart health.

Peanut butter

A more nutrient-dense ingredient to use instead of butter or oil in baking, peanut

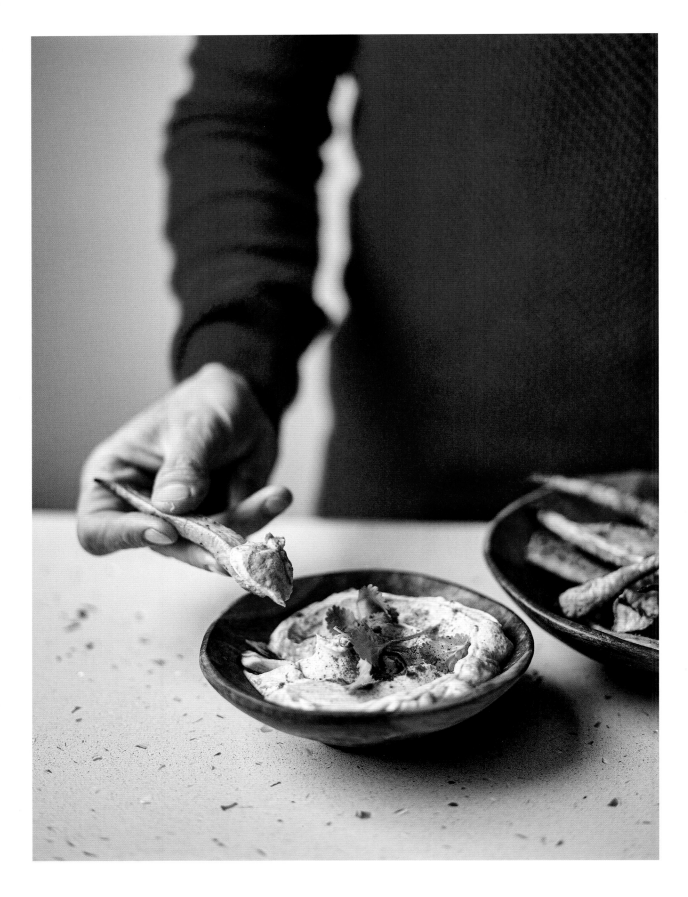

butter provides healthy fats, protein and fibre, which help control blood sugar levels and keep you feeling fuller for longer. It is also rich in vitamins E, B6, niacin, magnesium and phosphorus.

Potatoes (white and sweet)

Keep the skins on potatoes – they are super high in fibre, vitamin B and other nutrients. Cold cooked potatoes are even better for us (with low GI and higher levels of resistant starch). So, a cold potato salad contains more gut-loving fibre and promotes more slow-release energy. Sweet potatoes are full of beta carotene and a rich source of fibre. New potatoes are full of vitamin C and potassium.

Walnuts

These have been shown to have a calming

effect on the brain. Walnuts are a great plant-based source of omega-3 fatty acids (essential to our diets and good for heart and brain health) as well as other unsaturated fats.

Wholemeal flour

Wholemeal flour contains more micronutrients and is higher in fibre than white flour. Wholegrains are linked to better overall health and are a super important way to achieve the 30g per day of fibre that most of us should be aiming for.

JOE'S TIP

Remember, not all processed food is bad.

But do try to stick to lower-processed food. Fortified plant-based milks, tinned cooked beans and pulses, frozen veg, frozen berries, dried fruits, wholegrain pasta, wholegrain bread, tofu… these are all good elements of a balanced diet. Frozen fruit and veg, for instance, are great kitchen time-savers and have just as many nutrients as the fresh versions. Frozen blueberries have been shown to be even better than fresh, with higher levels of antioxidants. Using some processed foods can make it easier for you to meet your nutritional needs, so there is no need to cut them out completely.

DIETARY SYMBOLS

Vegetarian

Vegan

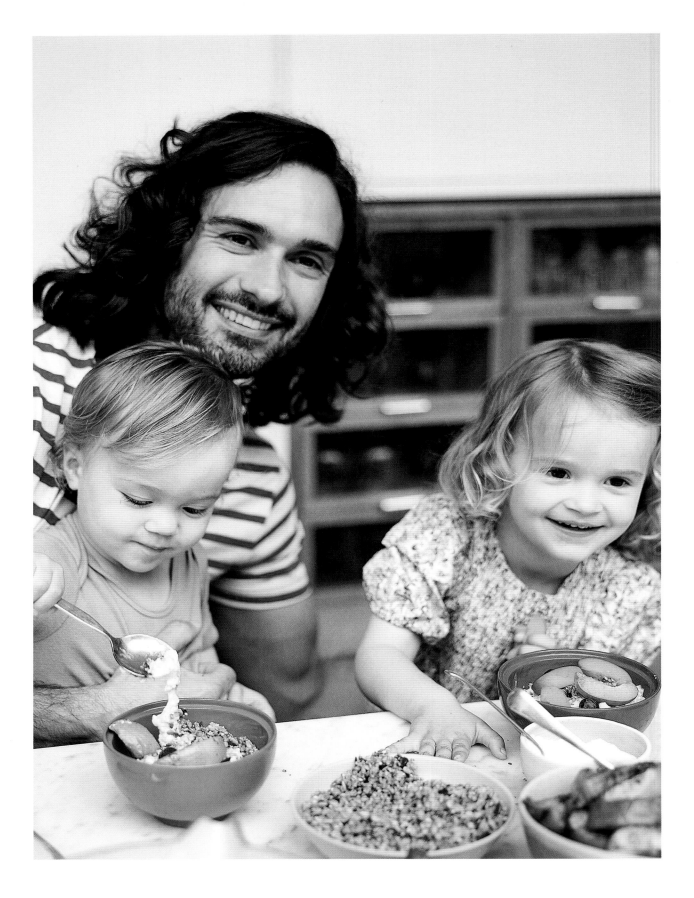

1

START RIGHT

breakfasts and brunches to help you wake up and power through

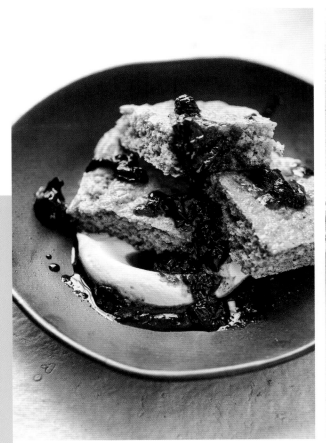

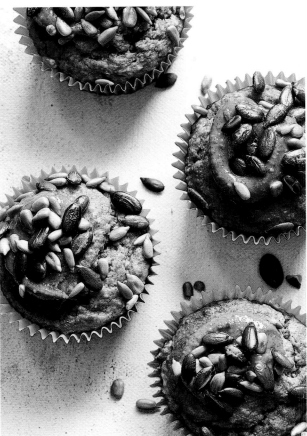

A good day starts with a great breakfast. A really tasty and filling meal at the beginning of the day sets me up for what's ahead – whether it's work or fun – and always puts me in a good mood.

It's a good idea to include some slow-release carbs, fibre and protein in your first meal of the day. This will help you control your blood-sugar levels for longer, so that you don't get a hunger crash mid-morning. All of the recipes in this chapter have that idea in mind and will help you power through to lunch without the need to start snacking.

I've tried to shake things up a bit with these recipes to give you some exciting new options to try. Whether you're in a hurry and need to grab and go, or

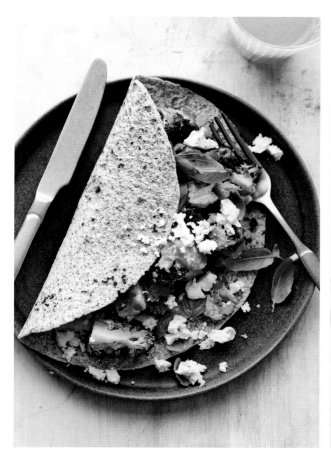

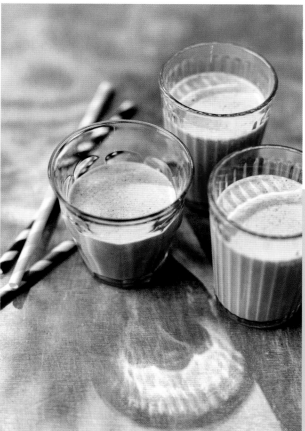

you've got the luxury of a bit more time to sit and enjoy a lovely brunch, you'll find something to suit. From super porridge toppings and tasty tacos, to eggy bread bakes or some creamy smoothies, I can't wait for you to taste them.

Pancakes have always been a favourite in my house, so it was a great day when I discovered a new easy way of cooking them. Baking the batter turns them into a cakey treat that may really surprise you. You'll find the recipe on page 42. There's also a recipe for good old crêpes, with some tasty chia jam for topping them off on page 46.

I'm so excited to share these recipes with you. Try them all – I know you're going to love them.

STRAWBERRY SMOOTHIE SURPRISE

The surprise in this smoothie is actually... cauliflower! Don't freak out and skip the page yet! Trust me, you can't taste it. It just adds more fibre and gives this smoothie a really nice, creamy texture. The banana and strawberry is what you'll really be tasting. It might sound strange, but give it a go and I think you'll be pleasantly surprised.

SERVES 2

200g frozen strawberries

2 ripe bananas, peeled

100g frozen cauliflower

1 tbsp smooth peanut butter or nut butter of your choice

200ml milk or non-dairy milk

1 Blitz everything together in a blender until smooth.

2 Divide between 2 glasses and serve.

JOE'S TIPS

- **Try using frozen blueberries instead of strawberries.**
- **You could also use coconut water as your liquid and frozen mango instead of the strawberries.**
- **Add a few tablespoons of oats or a scoop of unflavoured protein powder to make it more filling.**

FEEL GOOD FACT

Strawberries are a good source of fibre (for digestive health, gut health, helping to control blood sugar levels) and an excellent source of vitamin C (for skin health).

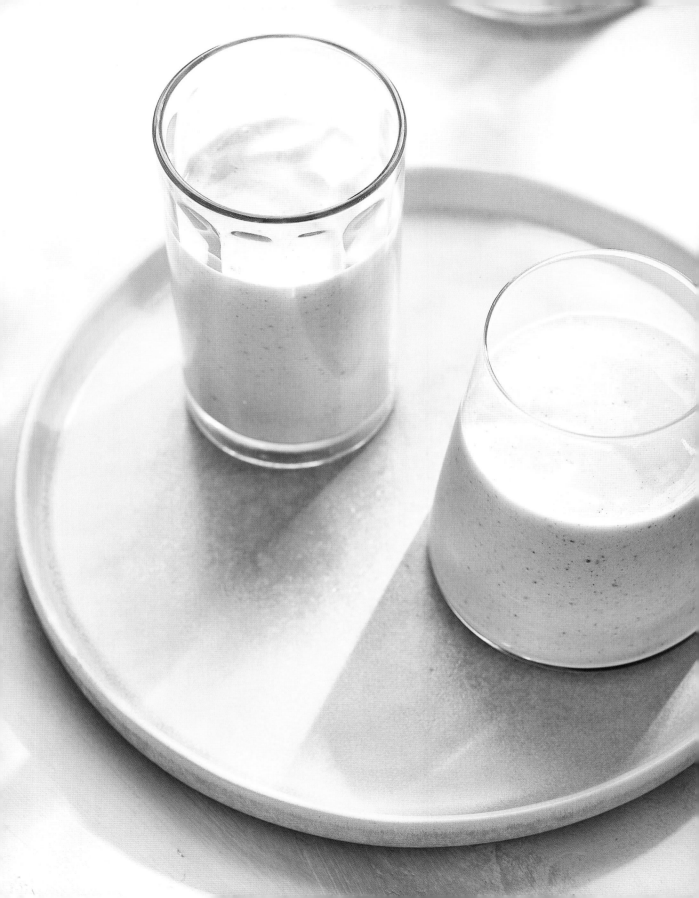

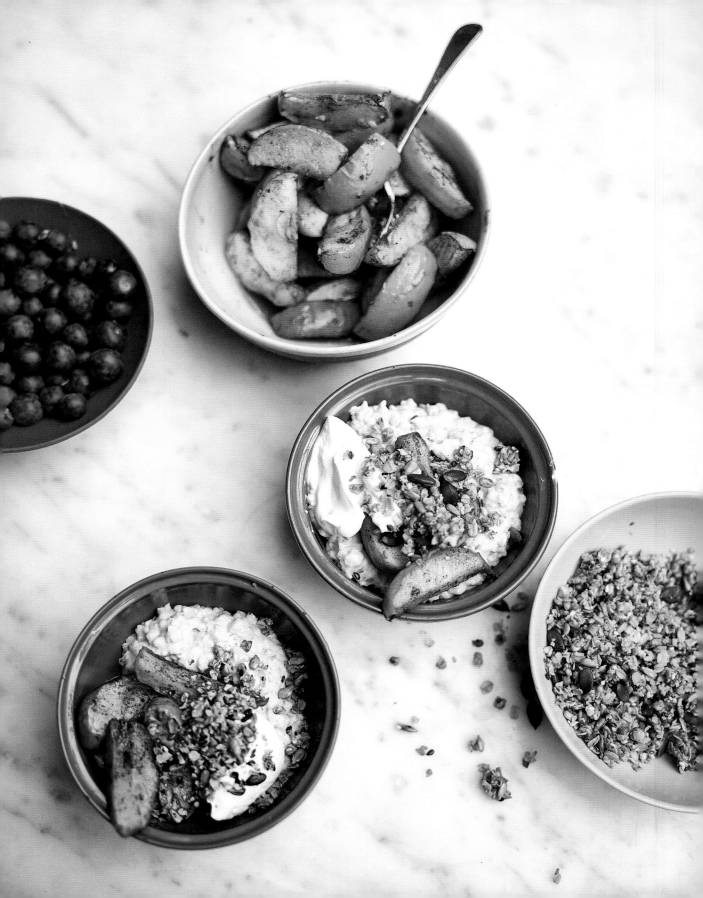

ROASTED SPICED APPLES WITH OATS – 2 WAYS

These cinnamon-spiced apples are so yummy, especially on top of your oats in the morning. Porridge is my go-to breakfast most days, as it's quick and healthy and such a great source of energy to start the day. I often add peanut butter, chia seeds or crushed nuts for an extra boost of healthy fats and protein. Here are summery and wintery versions, so you can mix it up your way.

SERVES 4

2 eating apples

zest and juice of 1 orange

1 tsp ground cinnamon

1 tbsp extra-virgin olive oil

1 tbsp light brown sugar or maple syrup

¼ tsp almond extract or 1 tsp vanilla extract (optional)

FOR A SUMMER TREAT:

Yoghurt Bowls with Toasted Oat Topping

5 tbsp porridge oats

3 tbsp mixed seeds (sesame, sunflower, pumpkin, flax, hemp)

2 tsp butter or coconut oil

1 tsp honey or maple syrup

300g low-fat Greek yoghurt

FOR A WINTER WARMER:

Whipped Porridge

500ml milk or dairy-free milk

450ml boiling water

160g jumbo oats

pinch of salt

2 egg whites

1 Preheat the oven to 200°C/180°C fan.

2 Core the apples and slice them into eighths.

3 Toss the apples into a roasting dish with the orange zest and juice, cinnamon, olive oil, sugar or syrup, and almond or vanilla extract (if using). Make sure they are well combined.

4 Roast for 30 minutes or until the apples are soft, stirring after 15 minutes. Serve warm or allow to cool, then pop into a lidded container and chill for up to 5 days.

For the yoghurt bowls with toasted oat topping

1 Toast the porridge oats and mixed seeds in a small dry frying pan over a medium heat until fragrant and starting to brown. Make a hole in the middle of the mixture and add the butter or coconut oil and the honey or maple syrup. Let it melt, then stir everything together until the oats and seeds are coated. Stir for another minute, then remove from the heat and allow to cool.

2 Divide the yoghurt between 4 bowls, top with the cooled roasted apples and the toasted oat mixture.

For the whipped porridge

1 Pour the milk and water into a medium saucepan and bring to the boil. Add the oats and salt, then bring back to the boil. Turn the heat off and cover with a lid. Let the oats sit for 5 minutes, then remove the lid, mix in the egg whites and turn the heat back on. Stir constantly with a whisk for 1–2 minutes until thickened.

2 Divide between 4 bowls and serve with the warm roasted apples on top.

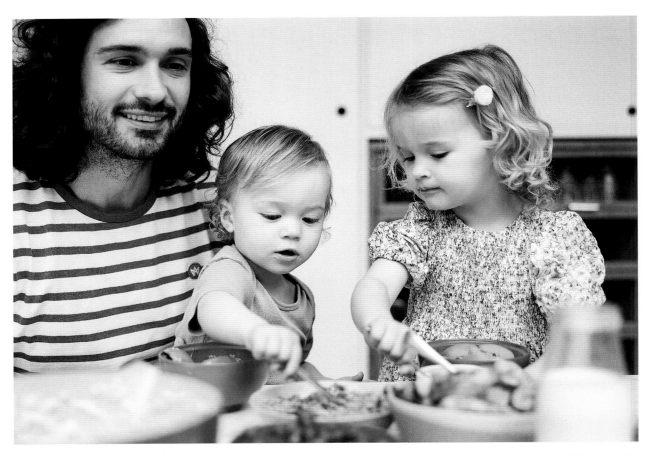

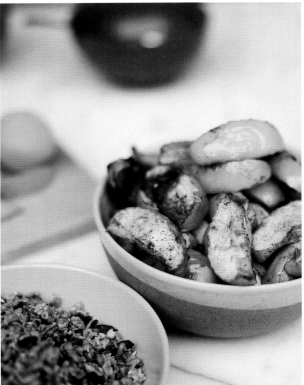

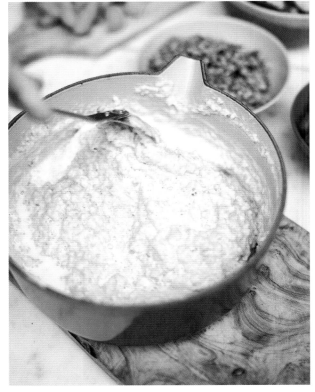

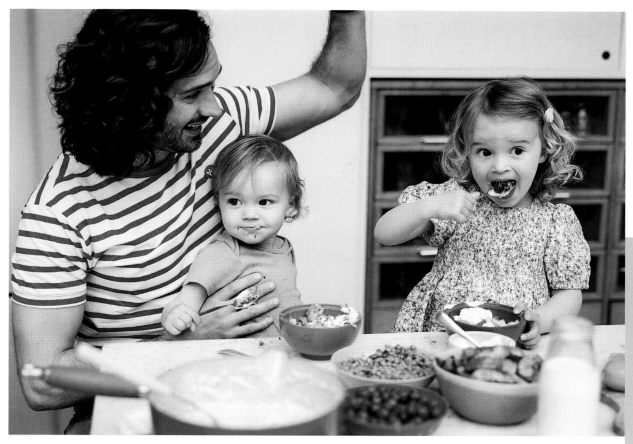

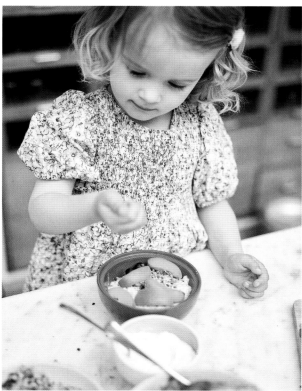

- Use pears instead of apples.
- Add a handful of frozen blueberries to the apples in the roasting dish.
- Add 50g roughly chopped dried fruit, such as dried figs, dried apricots or prunes to the apple mixture after it has roasted.
- Try lemon zest instead of orange zest.
- Add 1 tsp freshly grated ginger with the apples at the start.

START RIGHT

41

BLUEBERRY BAKING-TRAY PANCAKES

Everyone in my house absolutely loves pancakes for breakfast. It's good fun making the batter, flipping them, then adding all your favourite toppings. It can be a messy business, so this baking-tray version is much easier and quicker to make, especially when serving a big family of hungry little monsters. The batter is a bit thicker, so it's more like a cakey treat, and they taste incredible with yoghurt and this home-made blueberry compote.

SERVES 4

120g porridge oats

120g plain white or wholemeal flour

2½ tsp baking powder

¼ tsp bicarbonate of soda

½ tsp ground cinnamon

¼ tsp salt

120g natural yoghurt, plus extra to serve

120ml milk of choice

2 tbsp melted coconut oil or butter

1 tbsp sugar, runny honey or maple syrup

2 eggs

Blueberry Compote

250g frozen or fresh blueberries

1 tbsp lemon juice

1 tbsp granulated sugar

1 Preheat the oven to 200°C/180°C fan and line a 23 x 30cm rimmed baking tray (or a similar size tray) with baking paper.

2 Blitz the oats in a food processor to a coarse, mealy texture.

3 Tip the oats into a bowl and stir in the flour, baking powder, bicarbonate of soda, cinnamon and salt. Add the yoghurt, milk, melted coconut oil (or butter), sugar (or honey or syrup) and eggs and stir together just until you get a cohesive batter. Don't overmix.

4 Pour the batter onto the lined tray and spread it out into an even layer. Bake for 12–15 minutes until the pancake is set and a toothpick inserted into the centre comes out clean.

5 Turn the oven to the grill setting or preheat the grill while the pancake is baking. Transfer the tray to the grill and cook until the pancake is golden on top, around 1 minute.

6 Meanwhile, make the compote. Combine the blueberries, lemon juice and sugar in a small saucepan, cover with a lid and cook over a medium-low heat, swirling the pan occasionally, until the blueberries have released some juice and are soft. Remove from the heat.

7 Cut the pancake into 12 pieces. Pile 3 pieces onto each plate, top with the blueberry compote and a bit of yoghurt and serve.

JOE'S TIPS

- Instead of blueberry compote, you can top the pancake with fresh berries or sliced banana and a drizzle of maple syrup.
- Switch the cinnamon for the finely grated zest of ½ lemon or orange.

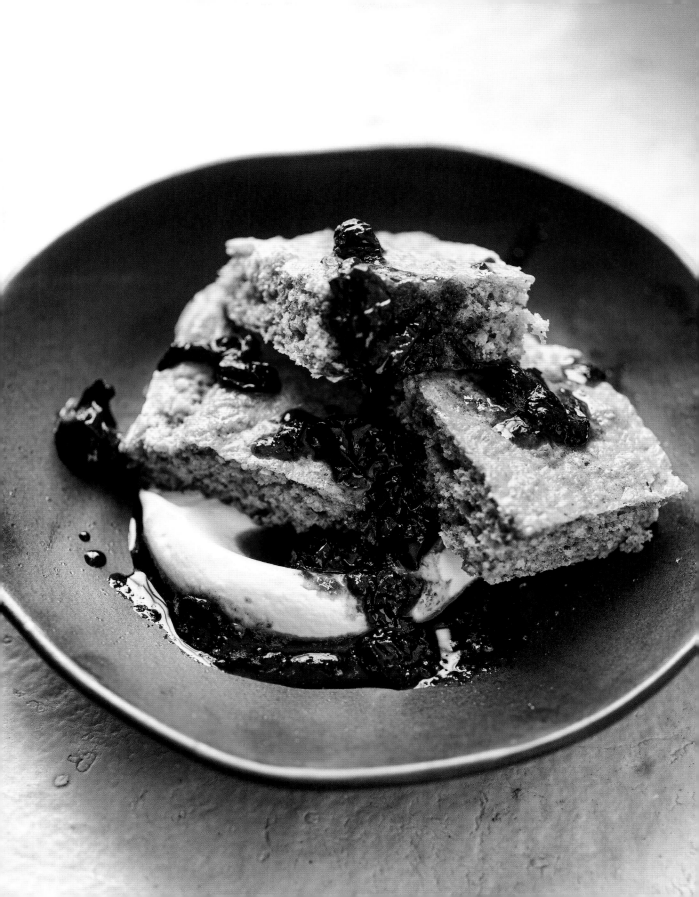

OAT & BANANA BLENDER MUFFINS

These oaty muffins will be a big hit with everyone in the house. They are perfect to eat hot for breakfast at home, or cold as a healthy snack on the go. They are sweet and fluffy and have lots of fibre and energy to fuel your body. It's a good way to use up any extra ripe bananas you have lying around, too. Enjoy!

MAKES 8

250g ripe bananas, peeled

100g porridge oats

50g ground almonds

1 tsp ground cinnamon

45g runny honey or light brown sugar

50g olive oil or melted coconut oil

2 eggs

1¼ tsp baking powder

¼ tsp salt

Suggested Toppings

peanut butter

fresh/frozen blueberries

chocolate chips

sliced banana

mixed nuts

mixed seeds

desiccated coconut

1 Preheat the oven to 200°C/180°C fan and line 8 cups of a standard muffin tin with paper cases.

2 Place all the muffin ingredients (apart from any toppings) into the jug of a blender. Blitz until you get a smooth batter.

3 Divide the batter among the muffin cups and sprinkle on any of your desired toppings that you would like baked in.

4 Bake for 25–30 minutes until a toothpick poked into the middle of a muffin comes out clean. Remove to a wire rack to cool (the muffins may sink slightly as they cool).

5 Once cooled, decorate with further toppings, as you like. They will keep in an airtight container for up to 3 days.

FEEL GOOD FACT

Oats contain beta glucan, a type of soluble fibre, which can help lower LDL cholesterol, leading to better heart health. Bananas contain potassium, which helps muscles contract, supports the function of the nervous system, aids digestion and helps regulate blood pressure.

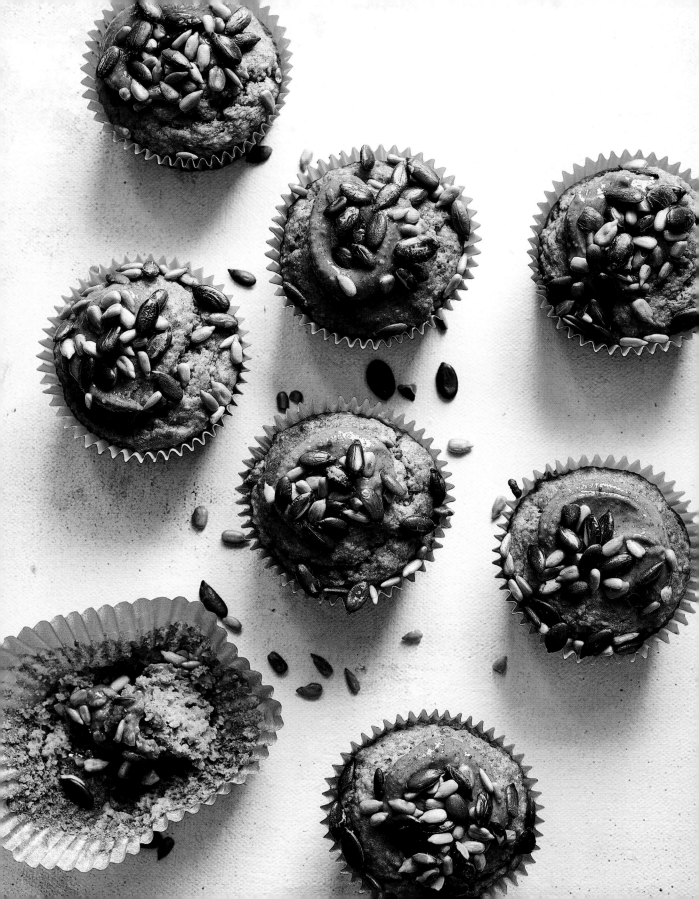

WHOLEGRAIN CRÊPES WITH STRAWBERRY CHIA JAM

Pancakes or crêpes? I couldn't choose a favourite if I tried, as I love them both. This recipe is a total winner because of the delicious home-made chia jam it comes with. It has such a lovely, sweet flavour and any leftovers can be used on toast, waffles, crumpets or scones. Win!

MAKES 12 CRÊPES

Crêpe Batter

60g plain wholemeal flour

90g porridge oats

4 eggs

320ml semi-skimmed or non-dairy milk

pinch of salt

2 tbsp melted coconut oil, plus a little extra for frying

Strawberry Chia Jam

200g frozen strawberries

1 tbsp runny honey

2 tbsp water

1 tbsp chia seeds

To Serve

low-fat natural yoghurt

1 Use a free-standing blender or electric hand blender to blend together all the crêpe batter ingredients until smooth. Leave to rest for 10 minutes.

2 Meanwhile, make the jam. Place the frozen strawberries, honey and water into a small saucepan and cover with a lid. Cook over a medium heat for 5 minutes until the strawberries have released some juice and have softened, then remove the lid and simmer for another 5 minutes to reduce slightly.

3 Use a potato masher or fork to mash the strawberries into a chunky paste (or blitz with a hand blender, if you prefer a smooth texture). Remove from the heat and stir in the chia seeds. Set aside to thicken and cool.

4 When ready to cook the crêpes, lightly grease a medium, non-stick frying pan with a thin layer of coconut oil and set over a medium heat. Pour in a few tablespoons of batter while tilting and swirling the pan to make a thin, even disc of batter. Cook until the underside is golden, then flip the crêpe over and cook on the other side. Remove the crêpe to a plate and set aside.

5 Repeat until you've cooked all of the crêpes.

6 Serve with the jam and some yoghurt on the side.

JOE'S TIP

You can store any leftover jam in a clean jar
in the fridge for up to 1 week.

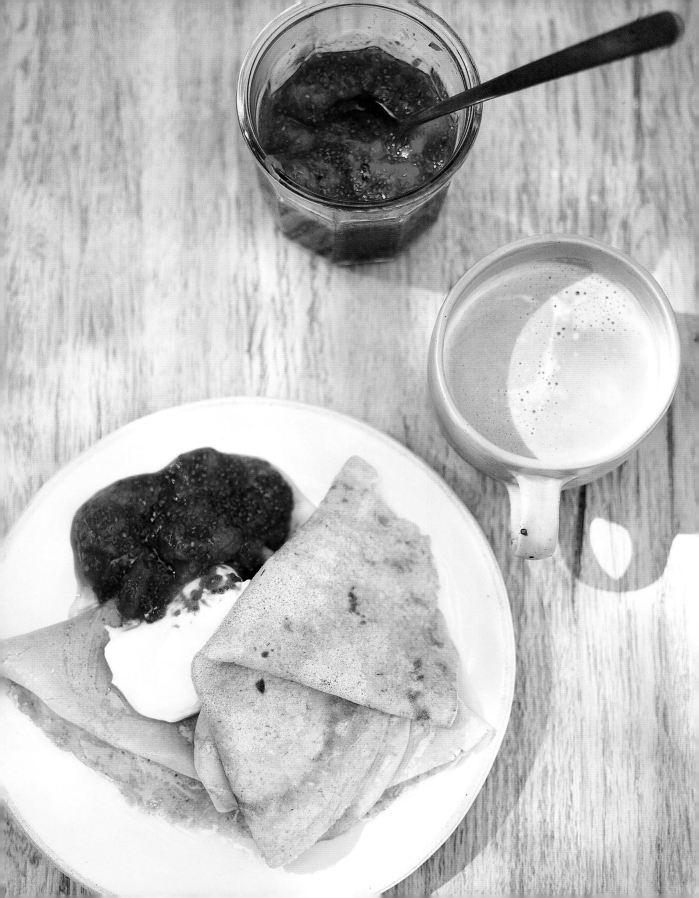

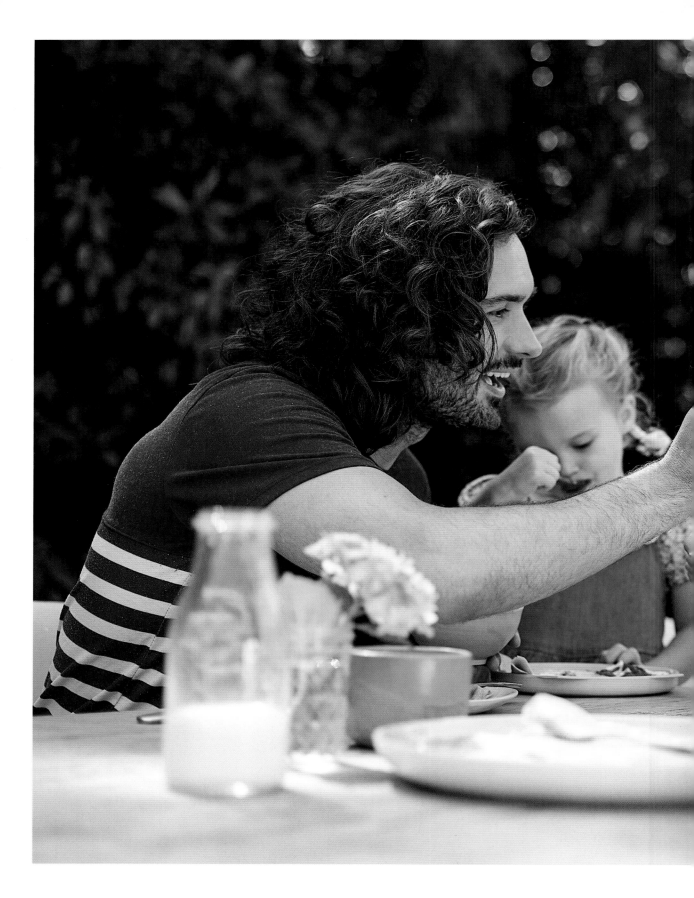

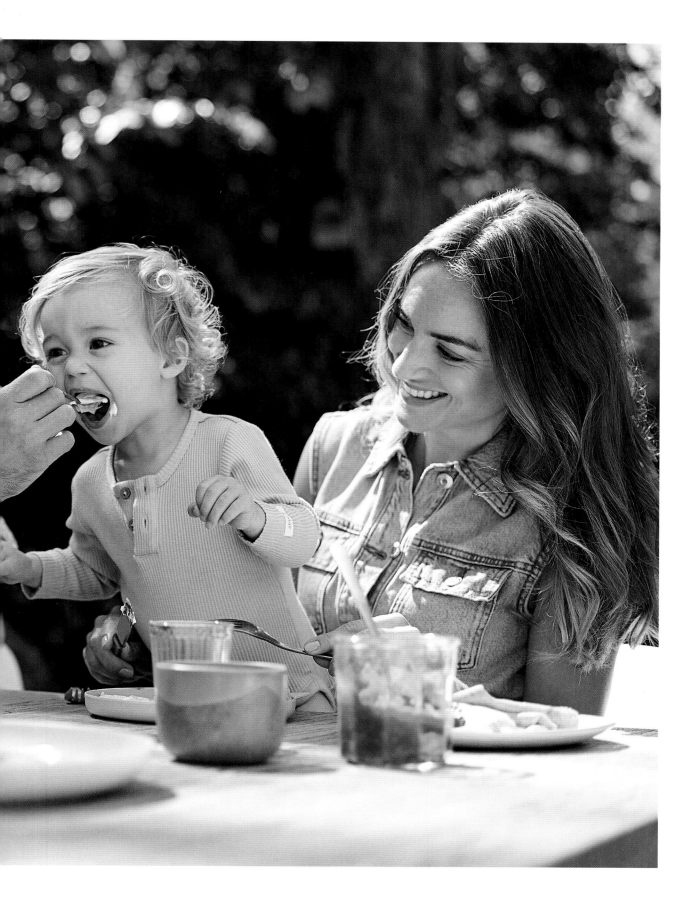

BAKED PORRIDGE CARROT CAKE

Carrot cake is probably my all-time favourite cake, so I said to myself, 'Why not turn it into a healthy breakfast?' This is the result. A yummy, baked porridge version with raisins and a crunchy seed topping. It's really easy to batch-cook for the family and can also be prepped ahead – keep it in the fridge and reheat whenever you want.

SERVES 4

light olive oil, for greasing

400ml milk or non-dairy milk

2 eggs

2 tsp ground cinnamon

¼ tsp ground ginger

¼ tsp ground nutmeg

¼ tsp salt

150g carrots, coarsely grated

200g porridge oats

100g raisins

50g mixed seeds

To Serve

natural yoghurt or milk

maple syrup or honey

1 Preheat your oven to 200°C/180°C fan. Lightly grease the inside of a 23cm square baking dish or tin (or one of a similar size) with a bit of olive oil.

2 In a large bowl, combine the milk, eggs, cinnamon, ginger, nutmeg and salt. Stir together until smooth, then add the grated carrots, oats and raisins and fold them all in.

3 Pour the mixture into the prepared dish or tin and sprinkle with the seeds.

4 Bake for 25–30 minutes, until the oats look set and dry on top but are still a bit soft in the centre.

5 Remove from the oven and cut into 4 squares. Eat warm with yoghurt or milk and a drizzle of maple syrup or runny honey.

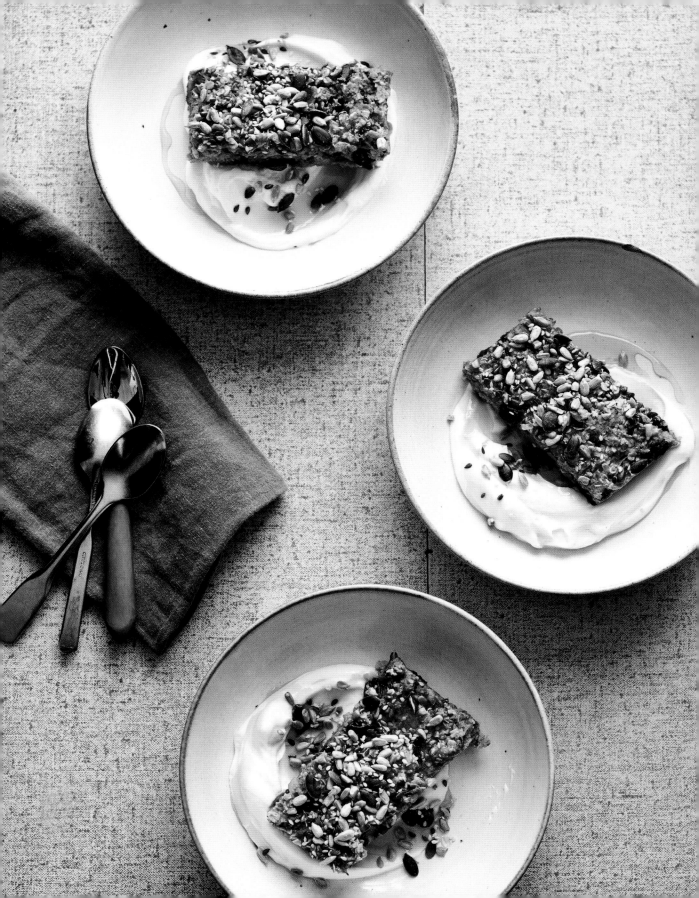

SCRAMBLED EGG & BROCCOLI BREAKFAST TACOS

Breakfast tacos are an awesome way to start the day, especially if you are busy and short on time. It's a super-quick way to pack loads of nutrients into your engine, too. Eggs are an easy-cook, cheap source of protein and healthy fat. In this recipe, I use broccoli and feta cheese, but you could really fill your taco with any veg you like, such as spinach, kale or peas.

SERVES 4

12 small tortilla wraps (preferably wholemeal or 50:50)

1 tbsp olive oil

400g frozen broccoli

2 garlic cloves, crushed

8 eggs

handful of basil leaves, torn

50g feta cheese, crumbled

salt and freshly ground black pepper

sriracha or other hot sauce, to serve (optional)

1 Warm your tortilla wraps according to the packet instructions.

2 Heat the olive oil in a large, non-stick frying pan over a medium heat. Add the frozen broccoli, stir to coat with the oil, then cover with a lid. Allow the broccoli to soften for 3–5 minutes, then remove the lid and continue to cook, breaking up any large pieces with your spoon, until it starts to brown.

3 Add the crushed garlic and stir in for 1–2 minutes to soften.

4 Whisk the eggs in a bowl with a pinch of salt and black pepper.

5 Remove the pan from the heat, pour in the eggs and stir through. Return the pan to a low heat and cook, stirring often, until the eggs are cooked to your liking.

6 Divide the scramble between the warmed tortillas and sprinkle with torn basil leaves and some crumbled feta. Drizzle with hot sauce, if using, and serve.

FEEL GOOD FACT

Eggs contain riboflavin (needed for eye and skin health, nervous system function and energy release), vitamin B12 (for maintaining a healthy brain and nervous system) and choline (important for nervous system function and cell building). Broccoli is a good source of fibre and is high in both vitamin K (needed for wound healing and bone health) and vitamin C (for skin health and boosting our immune systems).

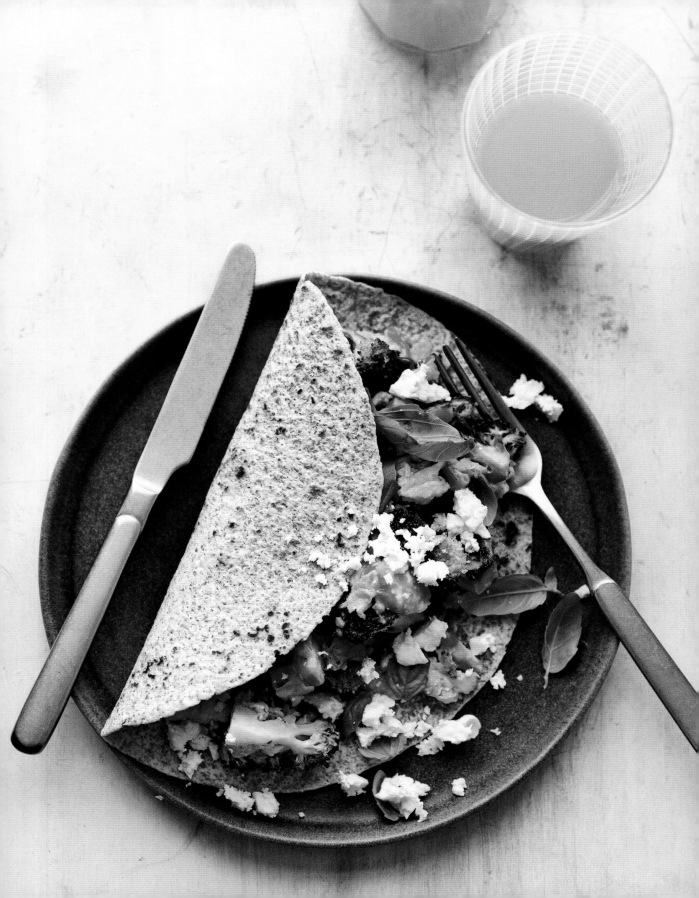

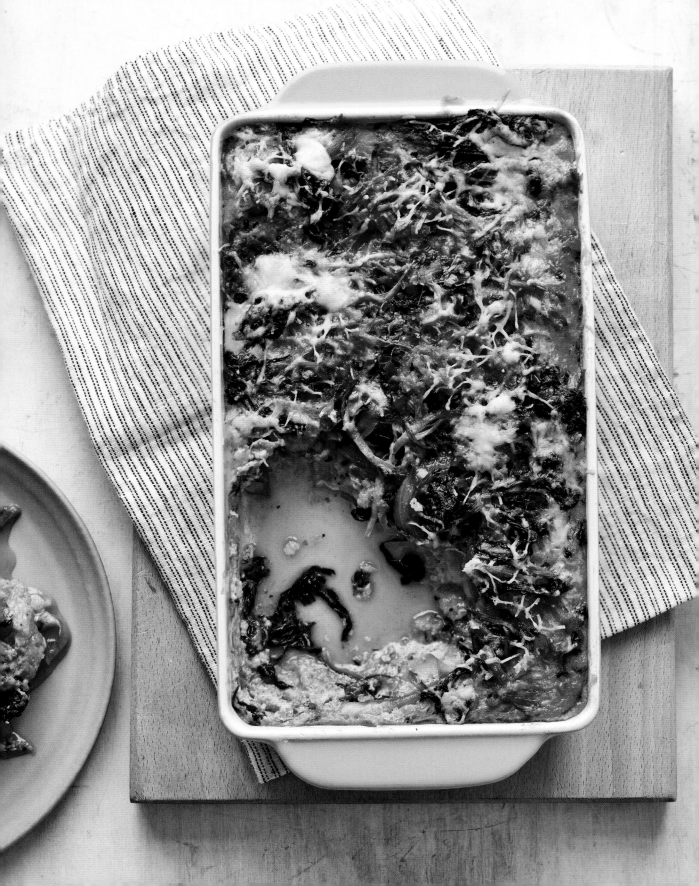

EGGY BREAD BAKE WITH SPINACH, HAM & CHEESE

This is a such a tasty recipe and a great way to get lots of extra veg into your breakfast. It's quick to prep and hassle-free, so if you have friends coming over for brunch stick this one in the oven. I'm sure they will all be asking for seconds!

SERVES 4

2 onions, sliced into 5mm slices

2 tbsp olive oil

1 tbsp balsamic vinegar

250g frozen whole-leaf spinach, defrosted

8 large eggs

500ml milk

2 tbsp harissa

4 sprigs of fresh thyme, leaves picked

400g crusty bread (preferably wholemeal), torn into 3cm chunks

100g shredded ham hock

80g Cheddar cheese, grated

salt and freshly ground black pepper

1 Preheat the oven to 200°C/180°C fan and line a 23 x 33cm (or a similar size) baking dish with a piece of baking paper.

2 Add the onions to a large, dry frying pan set over a medium heat and sprinkle with a pinch of salt. Cover the pan and cook for around 5 minutes, removing the lid to stir occasionally, until the onions are starting to brown. Remove the lid and turn the heat down to medium-low, then add the olive oil. Cook for a further 5 minutes, stirring occasionally, until the onions are nicely browned and soft. Stir in the balsamic vinegar.

3 Place the defrosted spinach in a sieve or colander set over the sink and squeeze out as much moisture as possible.

4 Add the spinach to the pan of onions and cook for a minute or so to dry the spinach out a little more, then remove the pan from the heat and set aside.

5 In a medium bowl, mix the eggs, milk, harissa and thyme with a pinch of salt and a good few grinds of black pepper.

6 Layer half of the bread chunks into the base of the baking dish. Top with the spinach-onion mixture and the shredded ham. Cover with the remaining bread chunks, then pour the egg mixture all over, aiming to soak all the pieces of bread. Finally, sprinkle with the grated cheese. Cover the baking dish with a sheet of foil.

7 Bake for 25 minutes, then remove the foil and bake for a further 20–30 minutes until set in the middle.

CREAMY MUSHROOMS, LEEKS & BEANS ON TOAST

Beans on toast is such a classic for me. It was the first thing I ever learned to make as a kid and I still love to make it now. Proper takes me back in time. This version is a bit more upmarket with the creamy mushrooms and leeks. I think you'll love the taste though and want to make this again and again!

SERVES 4

300g chestnut mushrooms, sliced

2 tbsp light olive oil

1 medium leek, cleaned and cut into 2cm pieces

2 garlic cloves, crushed

3 sprigs of thyme, leaves picked

400g tin of haricot beans

4 tbsp crème fraîche

1 tsp apple cider vinegar

4 slices of wholegrain bread, toasted

salt and freshly ground black pepper

1 Add the mushrooms to a large, dry frying pan with a pinch of salt and cook over a medium heat, stirring with a wooden spoon, until they've released all their liquid and are starting to brown. Add 1 tablespoon of the olive oil and cook until browned. Remove from the pan to a plate.

2 Heat the remaining oil in the same pan over a low heat. Add the leeks and a pinch of salt, and cook gently for 7–10 minutes until softened.

3 Add the garlic and thyme leaves and cook for 1–2 minutes.

4 Add the haricot beans along with their liquid and use the back of your spoon to roughly crush about a quarter of the beans. Stir through the crème fraîche, vinegar and cooked mushrooms, then taste and season with salt and pepper, as needed.

5 Top the toasted bread with the warm bean mixture and serve.

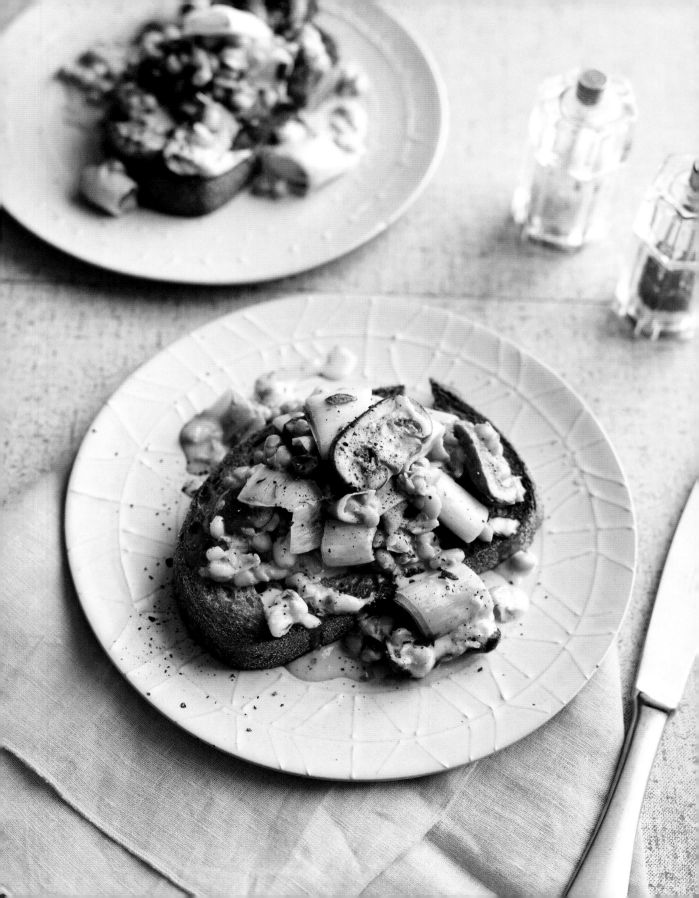

COFFEE & BANANA SMOOTHIE

This is one for the grown-ups who love a morning shot of coffee, although you can adapt it for kids by replacing the coffee with unsweetened cocoa powder (see Tip). It's a really yummy smoothie with a nice little kick to wake you up in the morning. It also makes a good pre-workout energy booster. You'll need to start your prep the night before, but it's so easy.

SERVES 1

1 ripe banana (or 150g frozen banana slices – see Tip)

1 tsp instant coffee

180ml milk or non-dairy milk

2 tbsp porridge oats

1–2 tbsp smooth peanut butter or nut butter of your choice

2–3 ice cubes

1 The night before, or a good few hours before you want to enjoy this smoothie, peel and slice your banana and place the slices on a baking tray. Freeze until solid.

2 When you're ready to drink it, simply add all the ingredients to the jug of a blender and blitz until smooth. Pour into a glass and serve.

VARIATIONS

- When very lightly sweetened, this reminds me of a frappuccino.
- You can add a splash of vanilla extract or a pinch of ground cinnamon for a flavour boost.
- Add 1 tsp unsweetened cocoa powder for a mocha smoothie.
- For kids: leave out the coffee and add 2 tsp unsweetened cocoa powder for a chocolate and banana milkshake.
- Protein boost: add a scoop of your favourite protein powder.
- For banana haters: use 150g frozen avocado flesh (pitted and peeled) in place of the banana – it'll make your smoothie super creamy! If you miss the sweetness of the banana, add a couple of pitted dates to your smoothie as well.

JOE'S TIP

Chop up extra bananas and freeze the slices on a tray, then transfer to a ziplock freezer bag. They will keep well indefinitely, but will be at their best for up to 3 months. You can then make smoothies whenever you fancy.

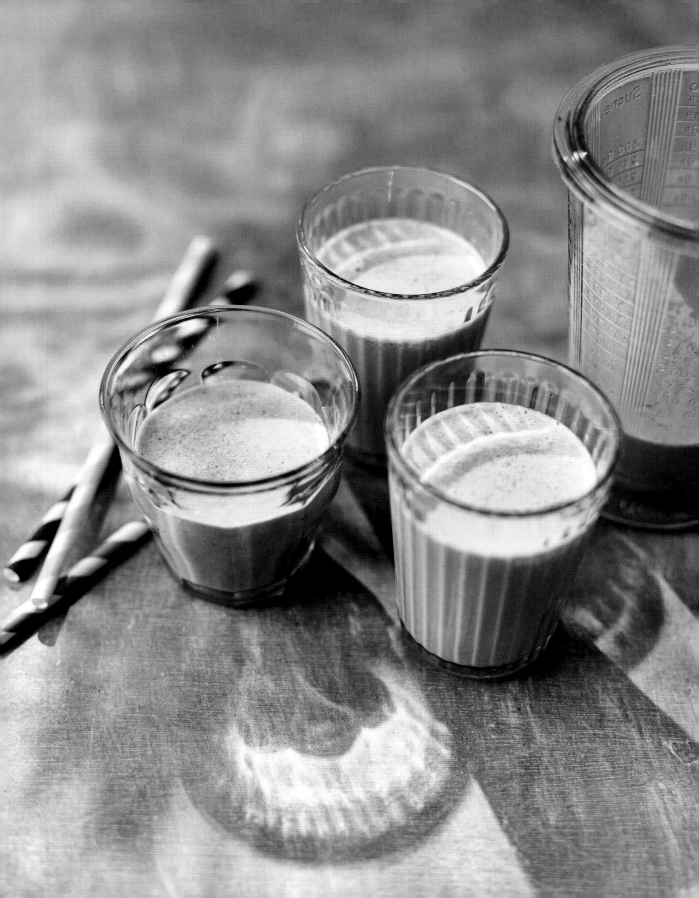

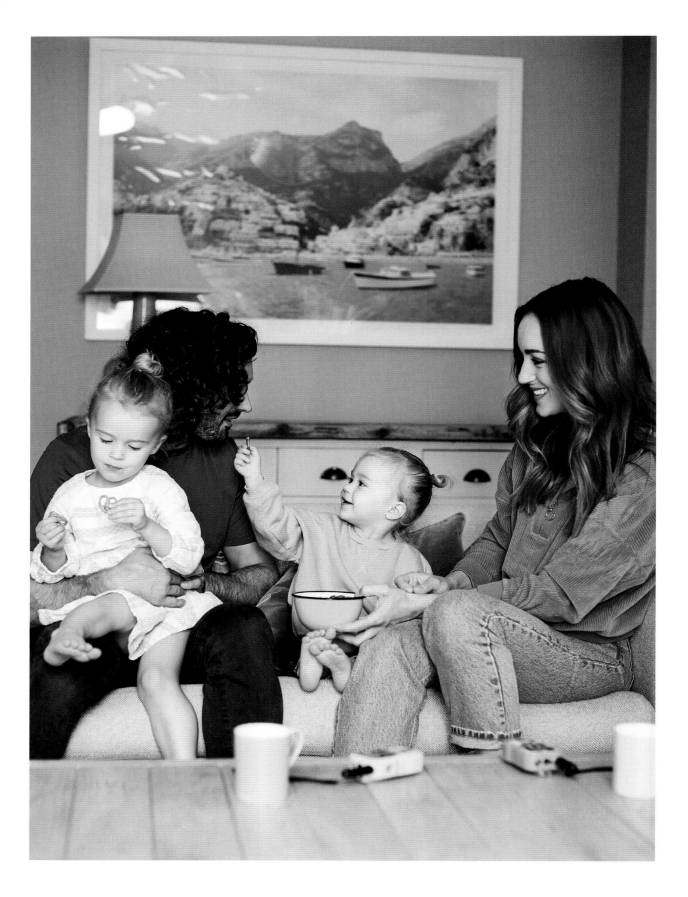

2

SNACK
SIMPLE

savoury dips and nibbles
to keep you satisfied

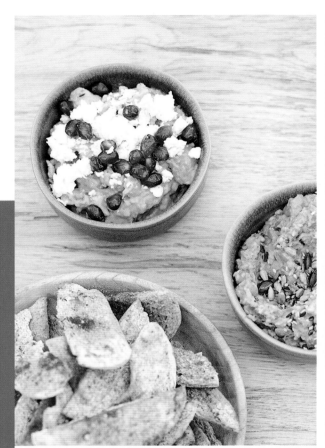

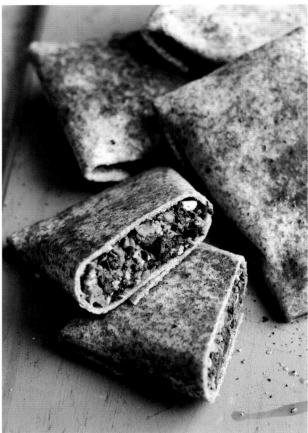

While it's a great idea to try to stick to three main meals a day and avoid unnecessary snacking, it's a fact of life that we all need a little boost from time to time. Not to mention all those occasions when friends or family come over and you need to offer up some tasty nibbles to keep everyone happy.

Whatever your snacking needs are, this chapter has got you covered. You'll find lots of new ideas for the classic chips-and-dips combo, plus some all-important post-workout or TV sofa session options.

When it comes to dips, I could never miss out on some hummus or guacamole action – they're simply the classics aren't they? So, to mix it up a bit, I've got some really fun ideas to give them a bit of a twist. Bet you never thought of

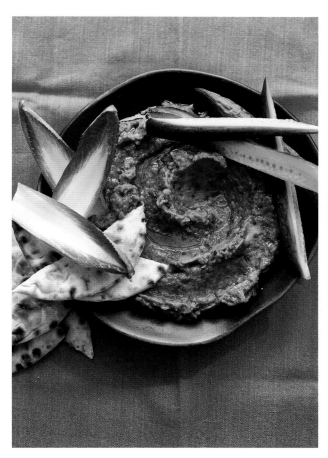

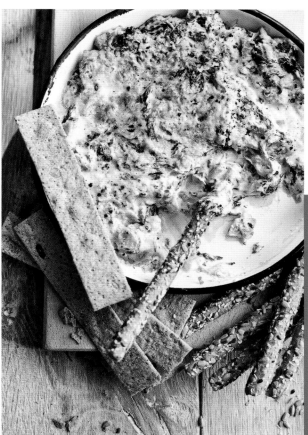

adding fruit to guacamole, but do – it's a taste sensation! There are loads of other ideas, too, from cheesy dips to spicy ones. I hope you try them all!

For dipping, try out my home-made chips (page 68). Made from tortillas or pita breads, they're a much healthier option than regular crisps or store-bought tortilla chips and are perfect for scooping up all the creamy dips.

Spicy, sticky baked nuts and pretzels (page 64) are good for those times when you just need to graze on something small. And for a more substantial option, try out the Turkish-style toasted wraps on page 84 – they'll certainly keep hunger at bay until your next main meal.

SPICY SMOKY NUTS & PRETZELS

Nuts and seeds are my number one go-to healthy snack. They are packed with healthy fats and are a great source of fibre and protein, which keep you feeling full for longer, so are ideal for a little graze between meals. If you find them too plain to eat on their own, spicing them up and adding some pretzels makes them much more interesting and tasty.

MAKES 8–12 SERVINGS

1 egg white

3 tbsp runny honey

1 tsp fennel seeds

2 tsp smoked paprika

1 tsp ground cumin

½ tsp chilli flakes

150g skin-on almonds

150g walnut halves

60g pumpkin seeds

30g sesame seeds

100g salted pretzels

1 Preheat the oven to 150°C/130°C fan and line a baking tray with baking paper.

2 In a medium bowl, whisk together the egg white, honey, fennel seeds, smoked paprika, cumin and chilli flakes. Fold in the nuts and seeds, then spread out in an even layer on the baking tray.

3 Roast for 20–30 minutes, stirring occasionally, until the nuts are toasted and the coating is dry (keep an eye on them so they don't burn).

4 Allow to cool, then stir in the pretzels.

5 Store in an airtight container for up to 1 week.

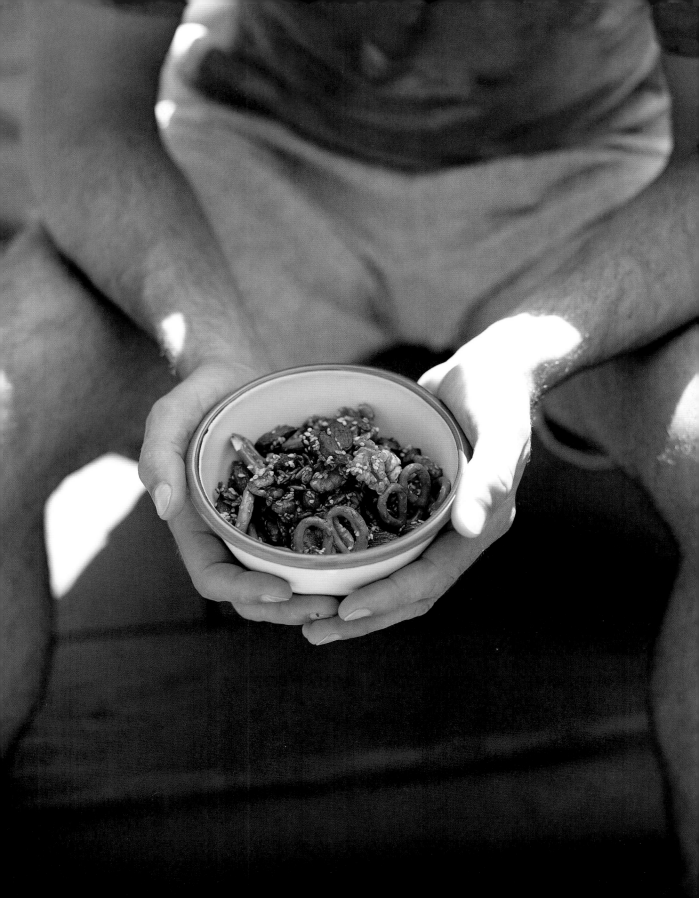

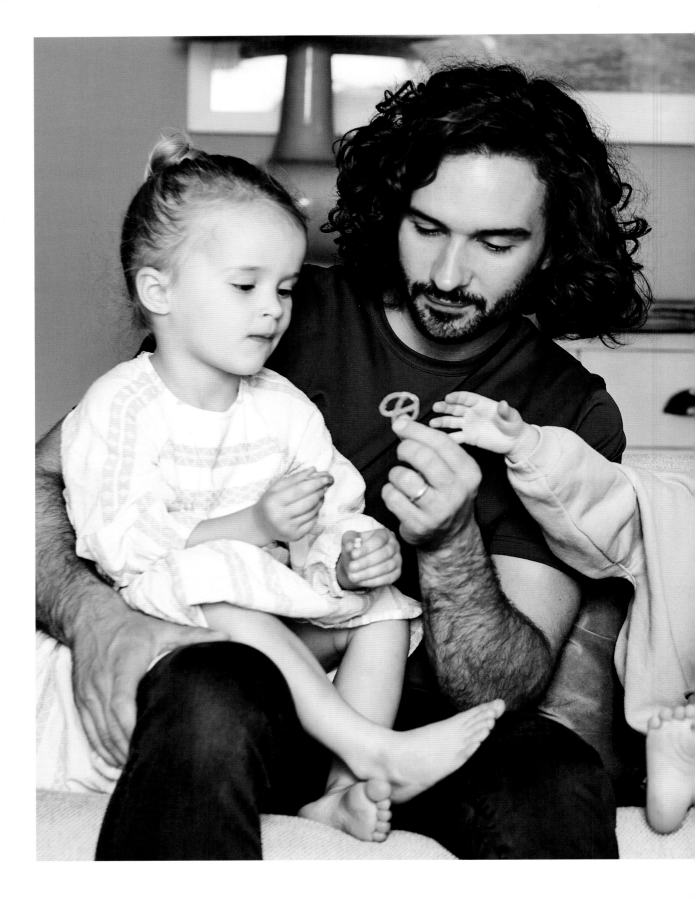

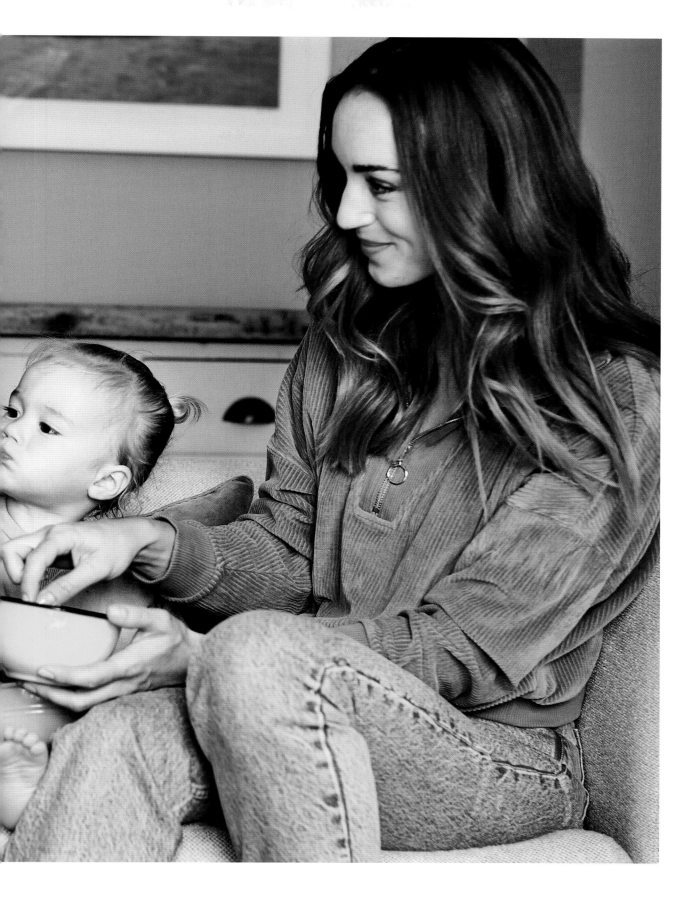

HOME-MADE TORTILLA OR PITA CHIPS

This is a super easy, quick way to make your own tortilla chips at home. They are ideal for dipping into all the dip recipes in this chapter, too. Baking them in a tiny amount of oil instead of frying them means they are much healthier than store-bought tortilla chips. Great thing is you can customise the toppings to make whatever flavour combos you fancy. I love using Cajun spice, smoked paprika, peri-peri or curry powder.

SERVES 2

2 large wholemeal tortillas or
  2 wholemeal pita breads
light olive oil, for brushing

Spice Mix 1

½ tsp smoked paprika
½ tsp ground cumin
pinch of salt

Spice Mix 2

½ tsp dried oregano
½ tsp garlic granules
pinch of salt

Spice Mix 3

½ tsp curry powder (or more if you like
  them hot!)
½ tsp nigella seeds
pinch of salt

1 Preheat your oven to 200°C/180°C fan.

2 For tortilla chips: use a pair of scissors or sharp knife to cut the tortillas into eighths. For pita chips: use a pair of scissors to remove the very edge of the pita bread, all the way around, then gently separate the pita so you have 2 thin ovals. Cut each oval into short strips, about 3cm wide.

3 Spread out the tortilla or pita pieces over a large baking tray.

4 Mix up your chosen spice mix, or all three, each in a small bowl.

5 Pour a little olive oil into a small bowl and use a pastry brush to lightly brush the tops of each chip with oil, then sprinkle the spice mix (or mixes) over the chips.

6 Bake the tortilla chips for 5–7 minutes until the edges of the chips are starting to darken. Pita chips will need 10–15 minutes until golden and crisp. You may need to remove any thinner chips earlier in the baking process, if they seem done before the thicker ones.

JOE'S TIP

You can easily double or triple the quantities here as needed.

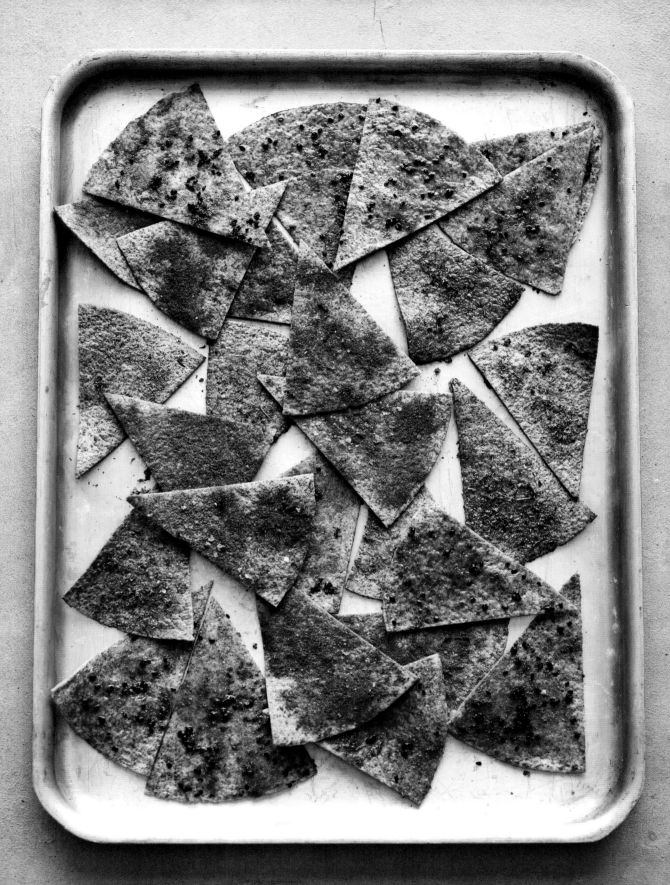

GUACAMOLE & VARIATIONS

If guacamole is good, then these variations are amazing! You might be surprised with some of the ingredients I've added, but give them all a try because they just work. The combination of flavours and crunchy textures are perfect with a tortilla or pita chip (see page 68), or vegetable sticks.

SERVES 4

2 ripe avocados

½ small red onion or 1 shallot, finely diced

75g cherry tomatoes, diced

handful of fresh coriander, finely chopped

juice of ½ lime

4 tbsp 0%-fat Greek yoghurt

salt, to taste

hot sauce, to taste

1 Cut the avocados in half, remove the pits and scoop the flesh into a wide dish.

2 Add the diced onion or shallot, cherry tomatoes, coriander and lime juice. Use a fork to roughly mash the avocado into a chunky paste.

3 Gently fold in the yoghurt, then season with salt and hot sauce, to taste. Serve immediately.

FEEL GOOD VARIATIONS

PEA & SEED

Defrost 120g frozen peas, then pulse in a food processor (or mash with a potato masher) until broken down but still a bit chunky. Stir into the guacamole in place of one of the avocados. Toast 3 tbsp mixed seeds in a dry frying pan until golden and fragrant, then tip out of the pan on top of the guacamole.

PEACH & BASIL

Replace the tomatoes with 1 ripe, diced peach. Stir in 2 tbsp chopped fresh basil along with the coriander.

POMEGRANATE, MINT & FETA

Stir in 2 tbsp chopped fresh mint along with the coriander. Garnish with a couple of handfuls of pomegranate seeds and 30g crumbled feta cheese.

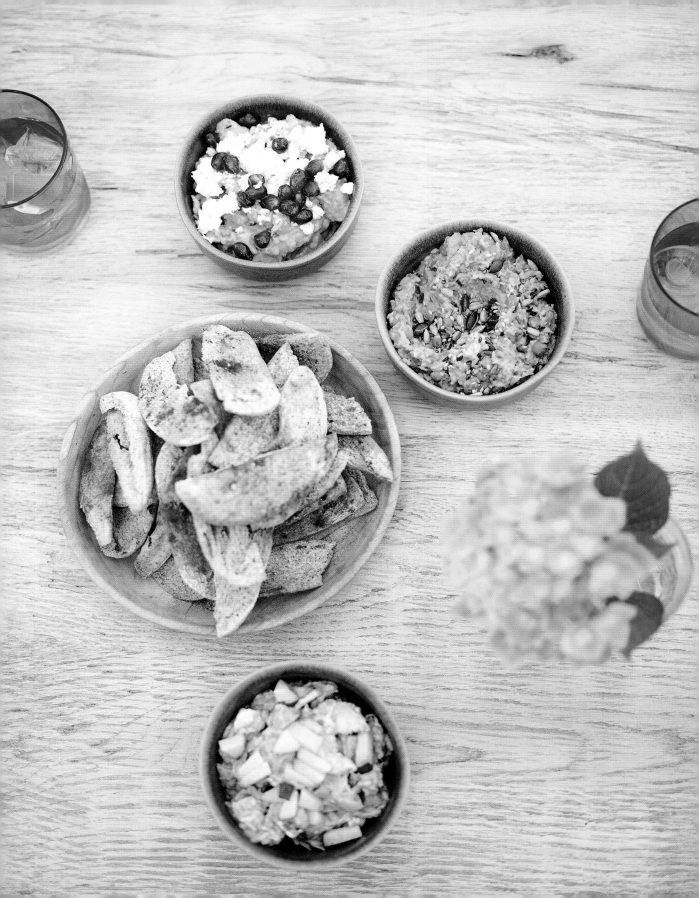

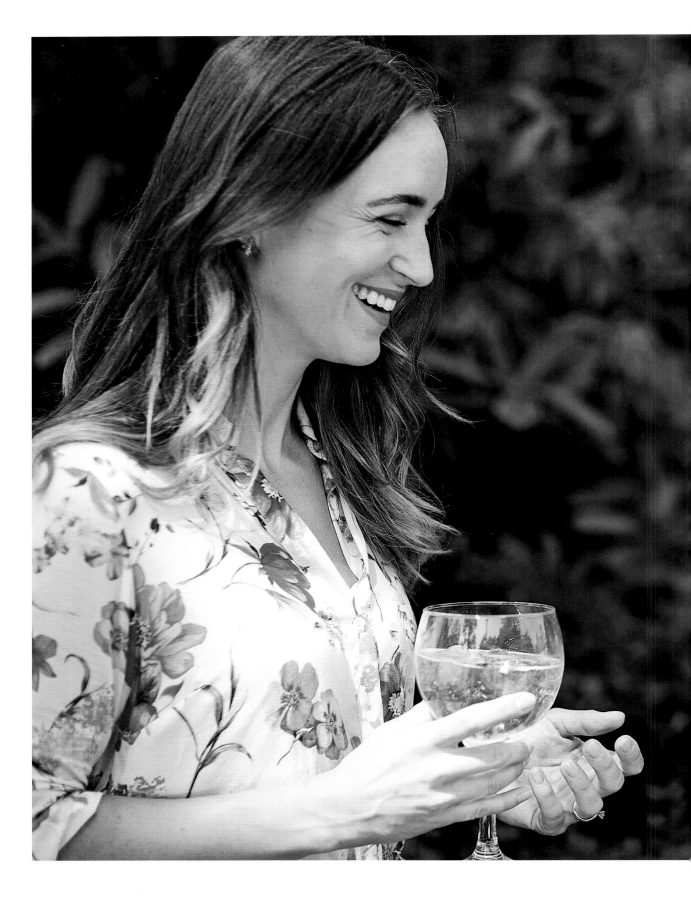

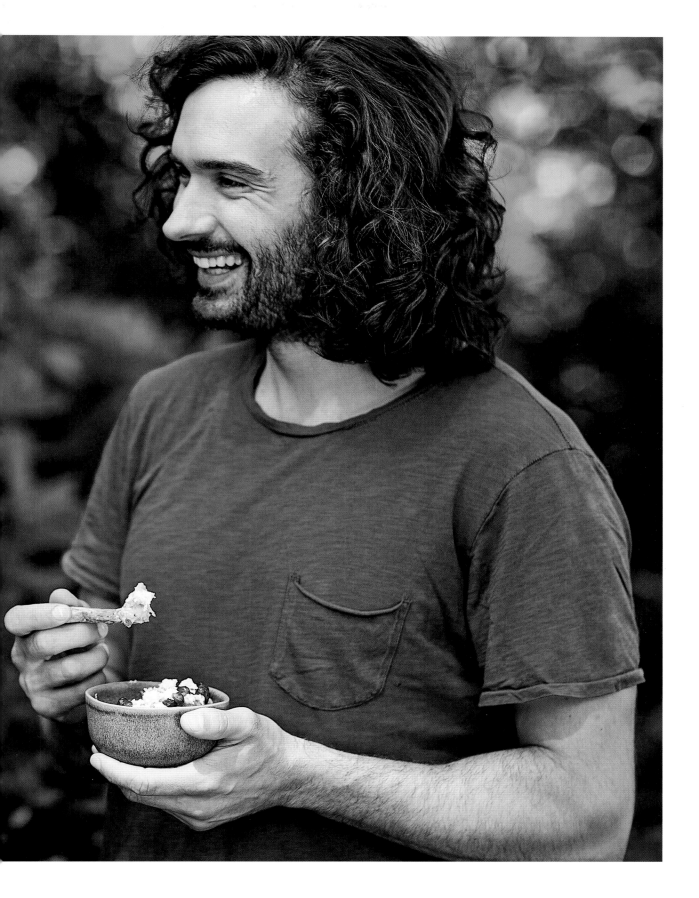

HUMMUS & VARIATIONS

Ve

Hummus always makes a great snack but it can taste a bit bland on its own sometimes. These four feel good versions I've created will take your chickpeas to a whole new level. More flavour, more texture and more crunch! Delicious.

SERVES 4

400g tin of chickpeas
1 garlic clove, peeled
juice of 1 lemon
2 tbsp extra-virgin olive oil
2 tbsp tahini
2 ice cubes
salt, to taste

FEEL GOOD VARIATIONS

PESTO & PINE NUT (V)
Replace the olive oil with 4 tbsp basil pesto. Toast 3 tbsp pine nuts in a dry frying pan until golden and sprinkle over the top of the finished hummus.

HARISSA & LEMON (V)
Replace 1 tbsp of the olive oil with 1 heaped tbsp harissa. Add the finely grated zest of ½ lemon and 2 tbsp of 0%-fat Greek yoghurt after you've blended in the ice.

MISO & WALNUT (Ve)
Add 2 tbsp white miso to the blender along with the chickpeas. Toast a handful of walnuts on a baking tray at 200°C/180°C fan for 7–10 minutes until fragrant, then roughly chop and sprinkle over the finished hummus.

1 Tip the chickpeas and the liquid from the tin into a small saucepan. Set over a medium heat and bring to the boil, then remove from the heat.

2 Meanwhile, add the garlic clove to a food processor or blender along with the lemon juice, olive oil and tahini. Blitz to chop up the garlic a bit.

3 Use a slotted spoon to transfer the chickpeas to the food processor or blender, leaving the liquid behind in the pan.

4 Measure out 60ml of the warm liquid from the pan and add to the food processor or blender. Blitz until smooth, stopping to scrape down the sides as needed.

5 Add the ice cubes and blend again until they've broken down and the hummus is light, smooth and the texture of natural yoghurt. Season with salt, to taste, then serve.

Note: If you prefer a thicker hummus, chill it before serving.

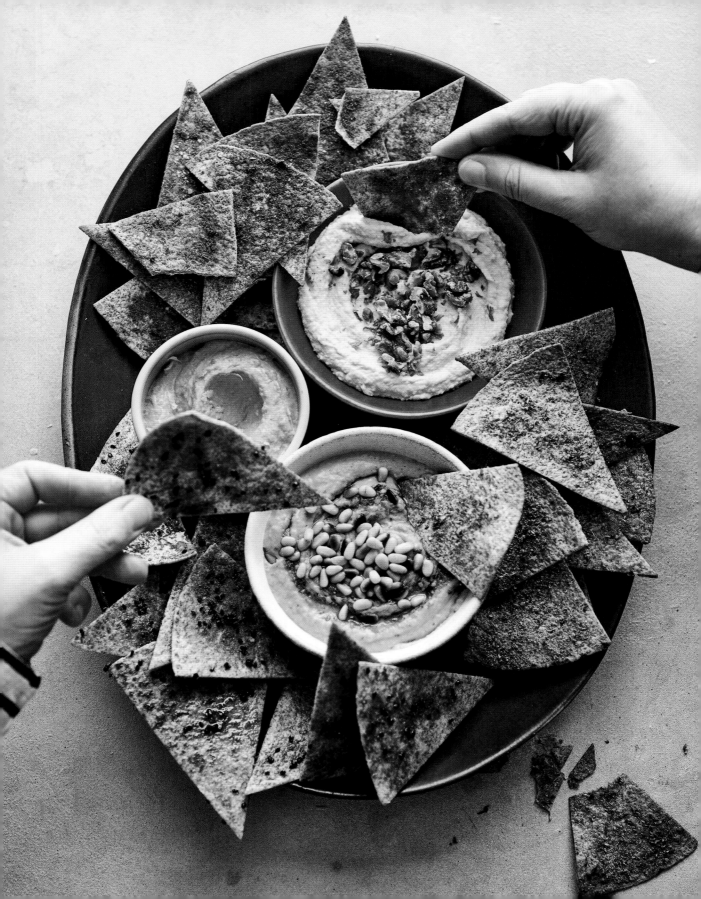

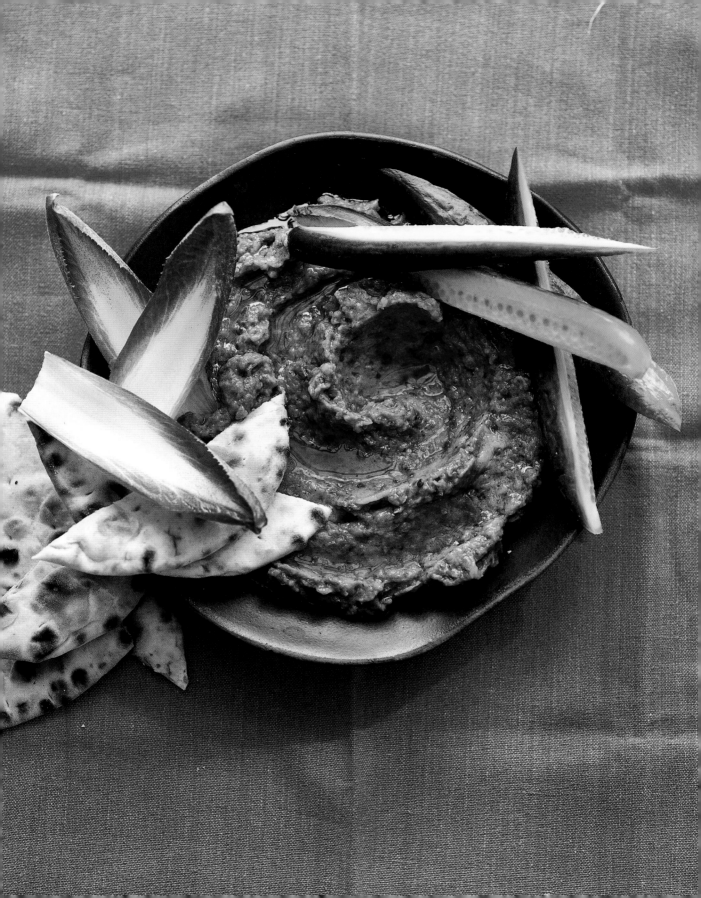

CREAMY AUBERGINE & SUN-DRIED TOMATO DIP

I'm such a big fan of mezze-style dips with bread, crisps or vegetable sticks. Back in the day, I would just buy pre-made dips from the supermarket, but when I started making my own it was a game-changer. The flavour and freshness in this with the roasted aubergine and sun-dried tomatoes is incredible. Defo give this one a go. It's worth the effort.

SERVES 4–6

1 aubergine

150g sun-dried tomatoes (packed in oil)

2 tbsp extra-virgin olive oil (or use the oil from the jar of tomatoes)

2 tbsp lemon juice

2 garlic cloves, crushed

salt, to taste

1 Preheat the oven to 200°C/180°C fan.

2 Prick the aubergine all over with a sharp knife and place it on a baking tray. Roast for 45 minutes–1 hour until the aubergine is super soft.

3 Once cool enough to handle, cut the aubergine in half, and scoop the flesh and of each half out into a food processor or blender (or a jug, if using a hand blender). Add the remaining ingredients, apart from the salt, and blitz until smooth.

4 Season with salt, to taste.

JOE'S TIPS

- This makes an excellent pasta sauce or pesto. You can dot it onto pizza, spread it onto tarts or eat as a dip with fresh veg and toasted pita bread.
- It freezes very well, so if you have any leftovers just pop them into a lidded container and freeze for up to 3 months. To defrost, let it thaw at room temperature until soft.

CHEESY ARTICHOKE & SPINACH DIP

Another day, another dip. This is a warm cheesy winner that everyone is going to want to polish off. If you've got a movie night or some friends coming over for drinks, then whip this bad boy up for the win. It won't last long.

SERVES 6–8

450g frozen whole-leaf spinach, defrosted

400g tin of artichoke hearts, drained and roughly chopped

250g ricotta cheese

125g ball of low-fat mozzarella, drained and roughly chopped

2 tbsp low-fat mayonnaise

20g vegetarian hard cheese or Parmesan cheese, finely grated

2 tsp dried oregano

3 garlic cloves, crushed

1½ tsp apple cider vinegar

pinch of freshly grated nutmeg

salt and freshly ground black pepper, to taste

To Serve (optional)

crudités

seeded wholemeal breadsticks or crackers

Home-made Tortilla or Pita Chips (see page 68)

1 Preheat the oven to 200°C/180°C fan.

2 Place the defrosted spinach into a sieve set over the sink and squeeze out as much moisture as possible.

3 Tip the squeezed spinach into a bowl with the remaining ingredients, seasoning with salt and black pepper to taste.

4 Tip the mixture into a 1-litre baking dish (or a similar size dish), level the top and bake for 25–30 minutes until the top is starting to brown.

5 Serve warm with crudités, crackers, breadsticks or home-made tortilla/pita chips (see page 70) for dipping.

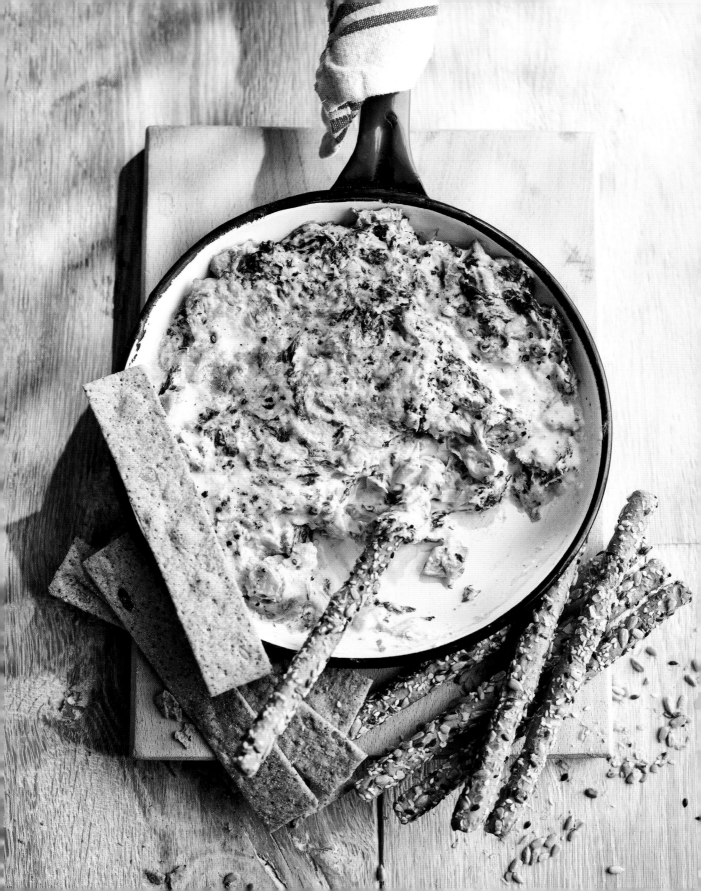

CHARGRILLED PEPPER, WALNUT & KIDNEY BEAN DIP

This recipe is based on the classic Middle-Eastern walnut and red pepper dip called *muhammara*. My version replaces the traditional breadcrumbs with kidney beans, which are packed with protein and fibre. It's really creamy and tastes amazing on some crispy bread or toasted pita.

SERVES 4

50g walnuts

280g jar of chargrilled peppers, drained

400g tin of kidney beans, drained and rinsed

2 tbsp apple cider vinegar

1 tsp ground cumin

2 garlic cloves, crushed

2 tsp smoked paprika

½–1 tsp chilli powder

2 tbsp extra-virgin olive oil

salt, to taste

1 Preheat the oven to 200°C/180°C fan.

2 Tip the walnuts onto a baking tray and roast for 7–10 minutes until golden.

3 Add the toasted walnuts to the bowl of a food processor and blitz briefly to roughly chop.

4 Add the remaining ingredients, apart from the salt, to the processor and blitz until you have a slightly chunky paste.

5 Taste and season with salt, as needed.

FEEL GOOD FACT

Walnuts contain omega-3 fatty acids, which are good for brain health, and have been shown to have mood-calming effects. Combining them with the protein and fibre in the kidney beans and the vitamin-packed red peppers means this dip is a proper superfood!

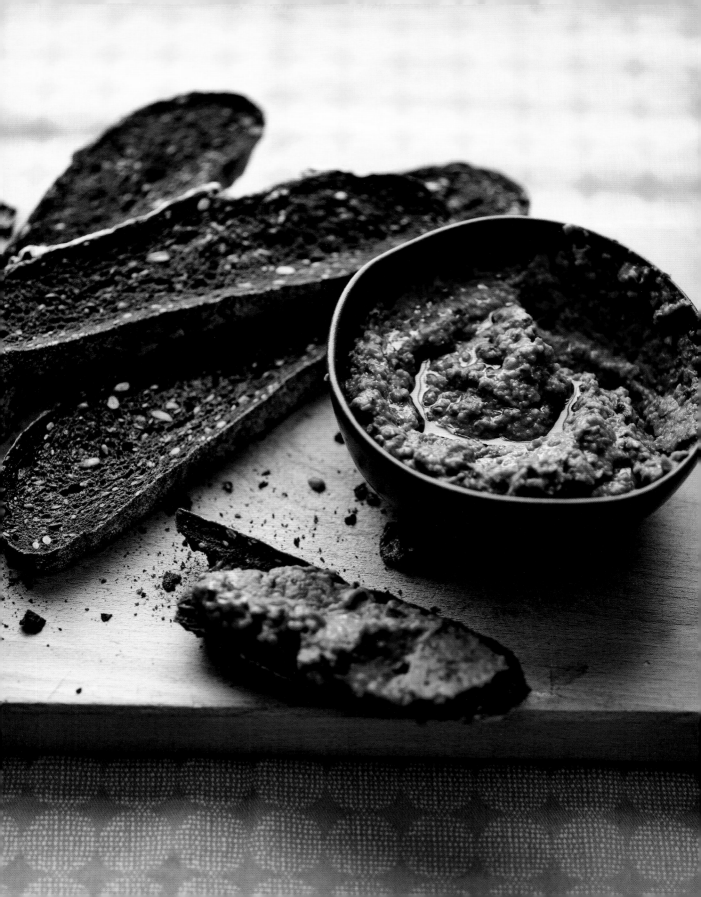

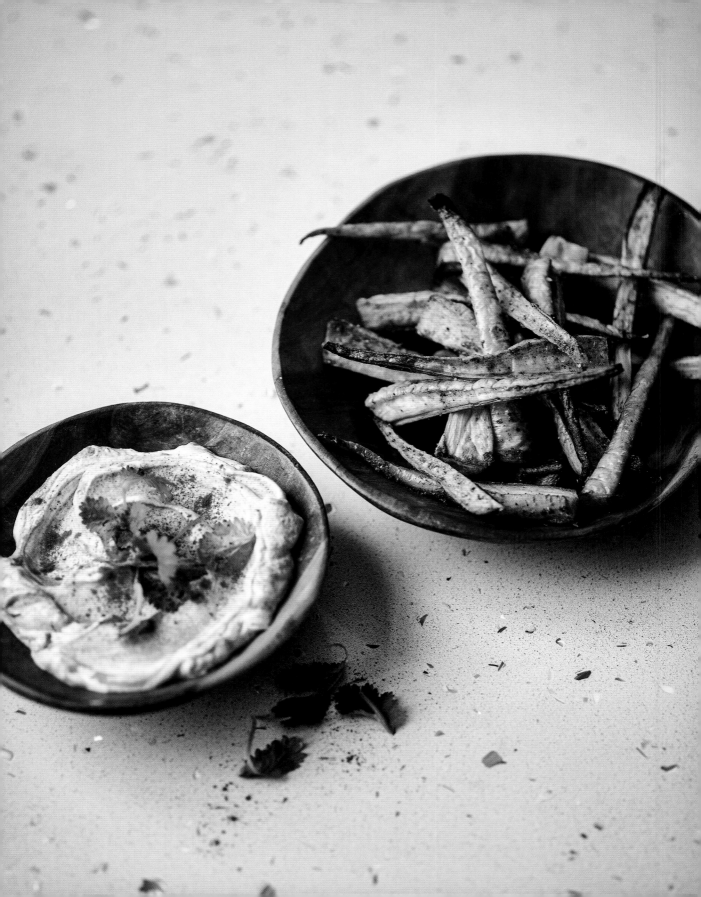

PARSNIP CHIPS WITH SMOKY YOGHURT DIP

Parsnips aren't just for Christmas or Sunday roasts! These crispy chips are awesome and so simple to make. This is one way I get Marley and Indie to eat more veg. They absolutely love them, especially with different dips.

SERVES 4

500g parsnips

1 tbsp light olive oil

½ tsp garam masala

pinch of salt

Smoky Yoghurt Dip

1 tbsp lemon juice

1 tbsp tomato purée concentrate (tomato paste)

½ tsp smoked paprika

pinch of salt

1 small garlic clove, crushed

4 tbsp low-fat Greek yoghurt

small handful of fresh coriander, roughly chopped

1 Preheat the oven to 240°C/220°C fan.

2 Cut the tops off the parsnips and slice them lengthways into halves (or quarters for bigger parsnips). Place on a baking tray and toss with the oil, garam masala and salt.

3 Roast the parsnips for 35–40 minutes until golden around the edges, flipping them halfway through the cooking time.

4 Meanwhile, make the dip by mixing together the lemon juice, tomato purée, smoked paprika, salt and garlic in a small bowl. Ripple in the yoghurt until just combined, then top with a sprinkle of fresh coriander.

5 Serve the dip with the warm parsnip chips.

JOE'S TIPS

- This also works with sweet potatoes cut into wedges, or carrots that have been quartered lengthways into skinny sticks, so use whatever veg is in season and available to you.
- You can thin the dip out with a bit more lemon juice and use it as a dressing on grain salads.

FEEL GOOD FACT

Parsnips are even higher in fibre than carrots and are a good source of vitamins C and K.

SNACK SIMPLE

CHEAT'S GÖZLEME

A gözleme is a Turkish flatbread that's stuffed with savoury ingredients and toasted. If you've never tried it before then you are in for a real treat. These use spiced mince and feta and are absolutely delicious. You can make them with veggie mince, too, to make them vegetarian. Usually, the dough is made from scratch, but it's so much quicker to cheat with ready-made wraps.

SERVES 4

1 tbsp olive oil, plus extra for brushing

1 onion, finely chopped

100g minced lamb or veggie mince

2 garlic cloves, crushed

½ tsp ground cumin

½ tsp ground coriander

½ tsp dried oregano

¼ tsp chilli flakes

250g frozen spinach, defrosted

80g feta cheese

4 wholemeal wraps

1 Heat the olive oil in a large, non-stick frying pan over a medium-low heat. Add the onion and cook for about 10 minutes until softened and starting to turn golden. Add the mince and cook until any liquid that it releases has cooked off. Stir in the garlic, cumin, coriander, oregano and chilli flakes and remove from the heat.

2 Place the spinach into a sieve set over the sink and squeeze as much moisture out of it as possible. Place the spinach in a medium bowl and tip the contents of the frying pan in too. Crumble in the feta and mix everything together.

3 Wipe out the pan with kitchen paper and return it to a medium-low heat. Take a quarter of the filling mixture and place it in the centre of a wholemeal wrap. Fold the sides in to meet in the middle, then fold the top and bottom in as well. Press down to form a rectangular parcel. Brush the wrap with a little olive oil and place seam-side down into the hot pan. Cook until browned underneath, then brush the top of the parcel with a little oil, flip and cook until the other side is golden brown. Repeat with the remaining wraps.

4 Serve warm, drizzled with a little more olive oil, if you like.

> ── FEEL GOOD FACT ──
>
> Spinach is rich in vitamin A (to support eye and skin health and immune function), folate (for forming healthy red blood cells, cell division, brain and nervous system function), manganese (to help certain enzymes function in the body, protect our cells from damage from free radicals, and to help form and maintain healthy bones), and vitamin K (for wound healing and bone health).

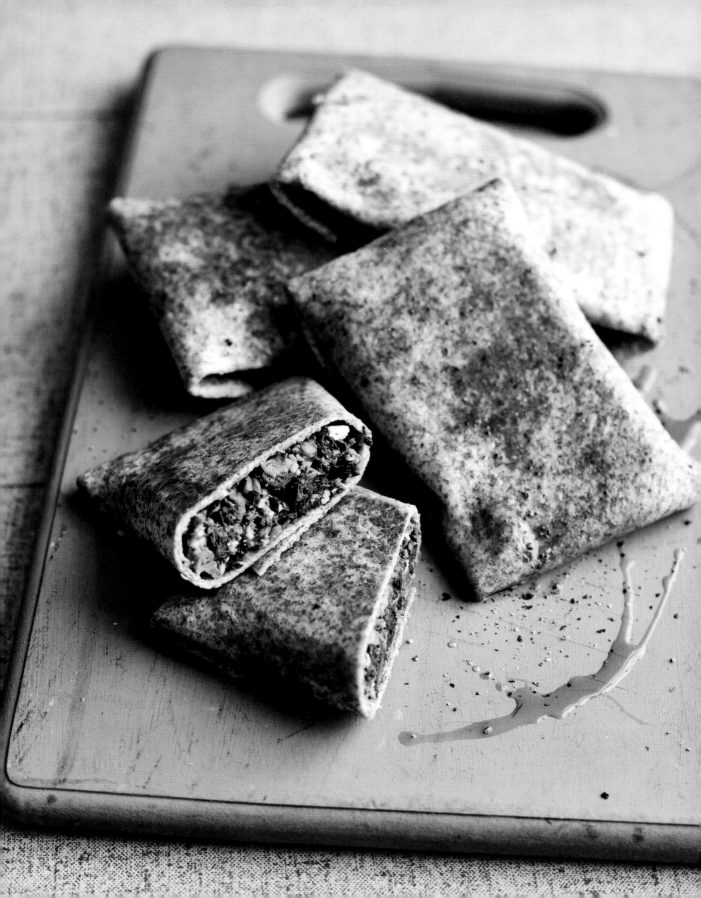

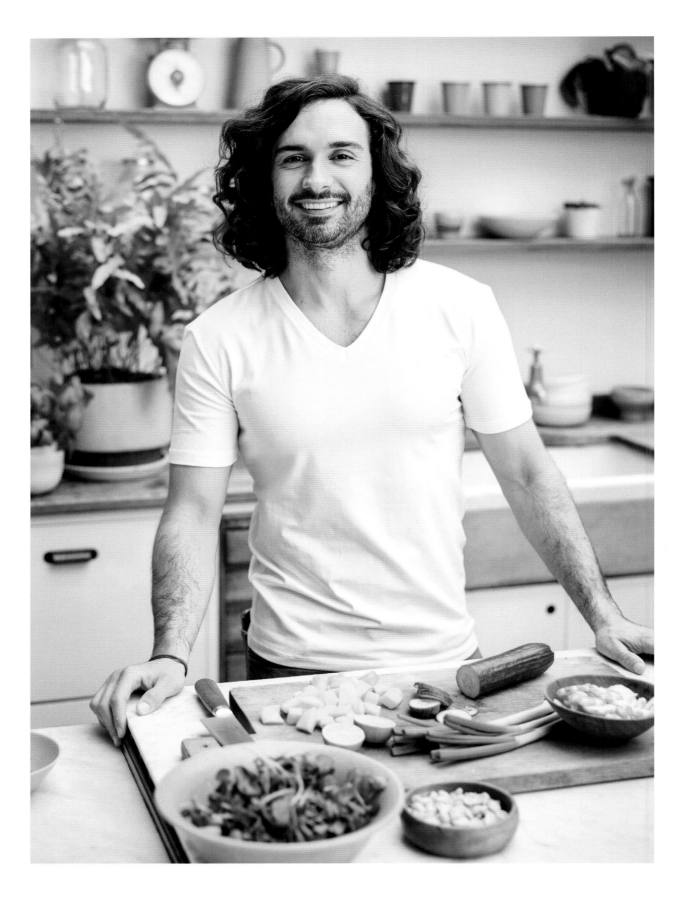

3

SMALL
BUT
SATISFYING

lighter meals and fun, fresh salads

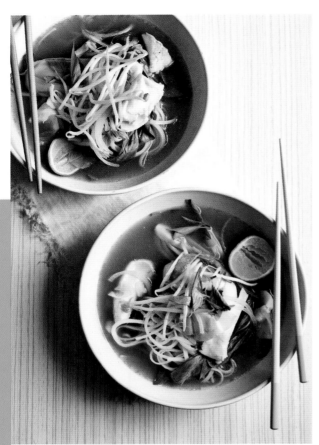
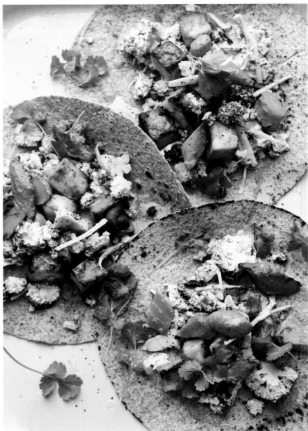

This chapter is packed with the most amazing salads and options for smaller meals – ideal for lunches, brunches or those occasions when you just want something a bit lighter.

As well as a fantastic, fresh collection of salads, you'll find some great wraps, fritters, a light, brothy soup and a super spicy rice bowl. I'm sure you'll return to these recipes again and again.

I don't know about you, but I sometimes feel hungry quite quickly after eating a salad, so my mission with these recipes was to make them really filling and full of fibre, so that you can feel properly satisfied after eating them. Every one is packed full of veg and all the vitamins you need to feel great.

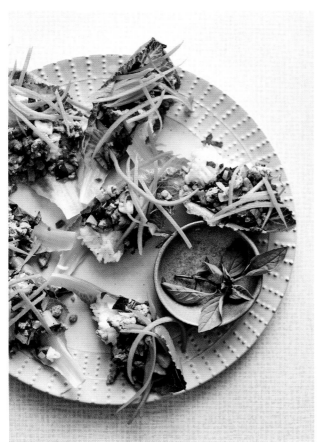

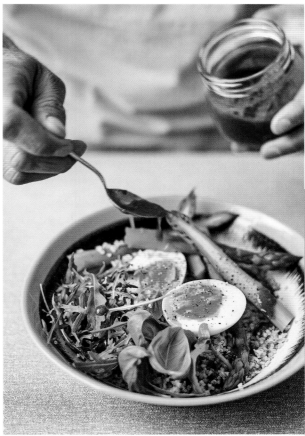

I've got some proper Wicksy specials in here – healthy twists on old classics, such as the Chicken Caesar Salad with Crispy Chickpea Croutons on page 107, my go-to Noodle Salad on page 92, and the most amazing salad dressings (such as the Peanut Dressing on page 92, the Herby Yoghurt Dressing on page 104 or the Miso Dressing on page 108) that can be used on so many other dishes to give them a flavourful kick.

Whatever style of food you're into, whether it's Mexican, Thai, Indian, Vietnamese, Japanese, Middle Eastern or Mediterranean, you're sure to find something in this chapter to send your tastebuds wild. The flavours in all these dishes are out of this world!

SPICED CHICKPEA, TOMATO & FETA SALAD

Sometimes you can be left feeling hungry again just twenty minutes after eating a salad, but not with this one. I always have plenty of tins of chickpeas in my cupboard as they're so versatile and cheap. They are rich in fibre and folate and are a fantastic low-fat, plant-based source of protein. They go so well with the feta cheese in this Mediterranean salad.

SERVES 4

1 tbsp cumin seeds

1½ tsp coriander seeds

juice of 1 lemon

3 tbsp extra-virgin olive oil

1 shallot or ½ red onion, thinly sliced

pinch of salt

400g tin of chickpeas, drained and rinsed

150g cherry tomatoes, halved

60g mixed salad leaves

50g feta cheese

10g (small handful of) fresh mint leaves, roughly chopped

10g (small handful of) fresh coriander, roughly chopped

1 tbsp pomegranate molasses or balsamic glaze

1 Toast the cumin and coriander seeds in a small, dry frying pan over a high heat until fragrant. Tip into a pestle and mortar and bash to slightly crush into a chunky powder (alternatively give them a quick pulse in a food processor or spice grinder).

2 Tip the spices into a mixing bowl, add the lemon juice, olive oil, sliced shallot or onion and a pinch of salt to the bowl and stir together. Tip in the drained chickpeas, cherry tomatoes and salad leaves and toss together.

3 Transfer the salad to a serving plate. Crumble over the feta, sprinkle with the herbs and drizzle with the pomegranate molasses or balsamic glaze.

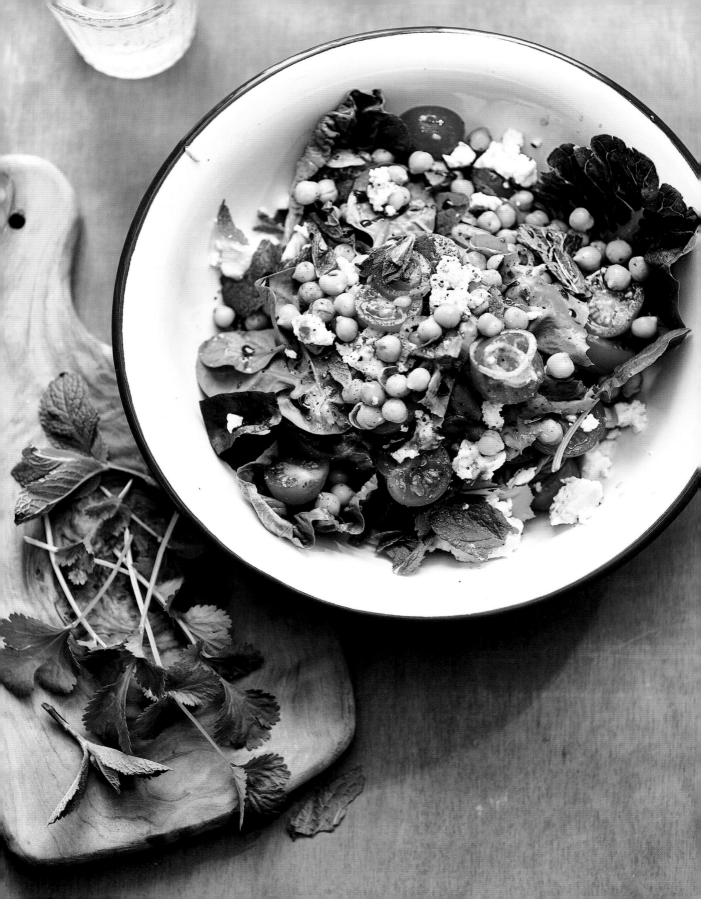

NOODLE SALAD WITH PEANUT DRESSING

There are not many things as simple and fast to make as this noodle salad. When I'm looking to make something quick at lunchtime, this is one of my go-tos. The nutty sauce tastes great cold, too, so this works well in a lunchbox on-the-go.

SERVES 4

250g dried egg noodles

2 tbsp sesame seeds

2 medium carrots, coarsely grated

½ cucumber, peeled into ribbons

4 spring onions, thinly sliced

1 red pepper, seeds removed, thinly sliced

handful of fresh coriander, roughly chopped

handful of fresh mint, leaves picked, roughly chopped

Dressing

3cm piece of fresh ginger, finely grated

1 garlic clove, finely grated

4 tbsp smooth peanut butter

2 tsp toasted sesame oil

4 tbsp soy sauce

2 tbsp rice vinegar

2 tbsp water

2 tsp runny honey

1 tbsp sriracha, or other hot sauce (optional)

1 Make the dressing first – simply whisk all the dressing ingredients together in a small bowl until smooth.

2 Bring a large saucepan of water to the boil and cook the egg noodles according to the packet instructions. Drain and rinse under cold running water, then leave to drain.

3 Toast the sesame seeds in a small, dry frying pan over a high heat until golden and fragrant. Set aside to cool.

4 Tip all the prepped vegetables into a large bowl, then add the noodles and dressing. Toss together until everything is nicely coated, then divide among 4 bowls or plates. Top with the toasted sesame seeds, the fresh coriander and mint.

JOE'S TIPS

- For a vegetarian protein boost, add frozen podded edamame beans to the pot of noodles as they cook.
- Add cooked prawns or shredded leftover roast chicken, to make it more substantial.
- Use different seasonal raw vegetables: finely sliced green or red cabbage, sugar snap peas, courgette peeled into ribbons, beansprouts...
- You can use almond butter or tahini in place of the peanut butter if you have a peanut allergy.

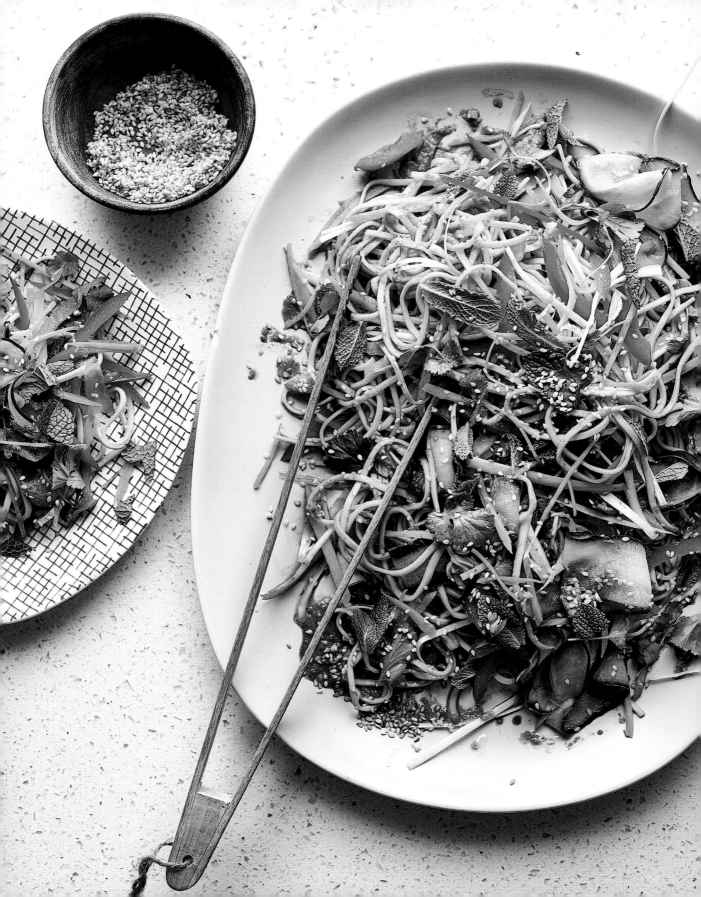

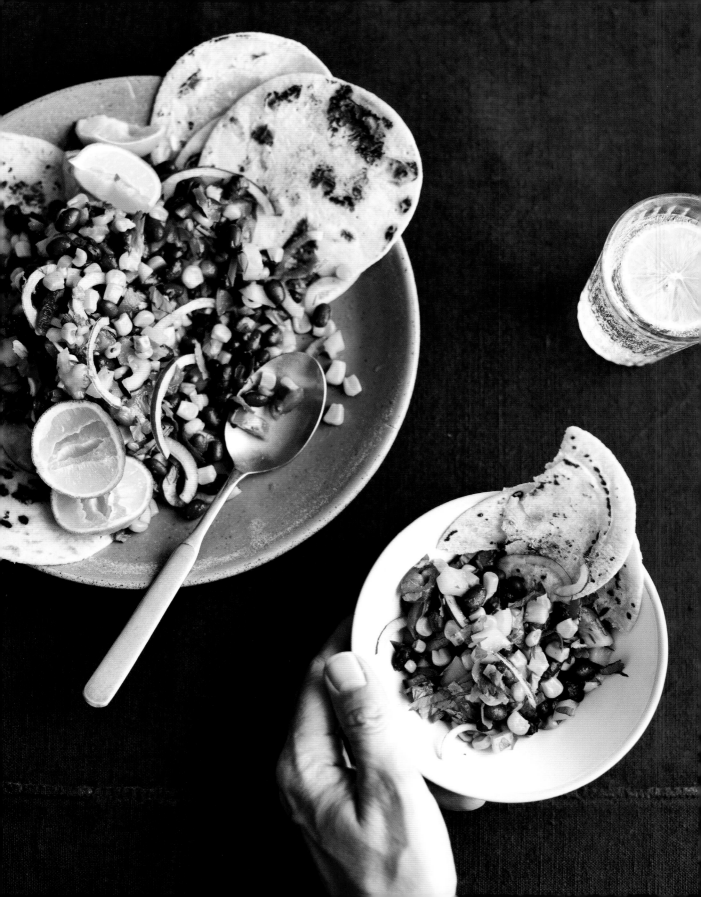

BLACK BEAN, CORN & JALAPEÑO SALAD

This colourful salad is super simple to throw together, with minimal prep. It's perfect on it's own or as a yummy veg-packed side to add to a main meal. It works really well with Mexican food, too. It's fresh, healthy and full of flavour. Enjoy!

SERVES 4

300g frozen sweetcorn

2 tbsp extra-virgin olive oil

400g plum tomatoes, diced

400g tin of black beans, drained and rinsed

1 red pepper, seeds removed, diced

½ red onion, thinly sliced

2 tbsp pickled jalapeños, roughly chopped

2 tbsp lime juice, plus extra lime wedges for serving

pinch of salt

handful of fresh coriander, roughly chopped

flatbreads, warmed, to serve (optional)

1 Add the frozen sweetcorn to a large frying pan with 1 tablespoon of the oil. Fry over a high heat until the corn is starting to brown, then add the diced tomatoes and cook for a minute more to soften slightly.

2 Tip the corn and tomato mixture into a bowl and stir in the black beans, pepper, onion and jalapeños. Dress with the remaining olive oil, the lime juice and salt.

3 Serve, scattered with the coriander, with extra lime wedges on the side for squeezing over. I like to scoop it up with some warm flatbreads, but it's up to you.

PEACH & BASIL PANZANELLA

This Italian-style salad with crunchy croutons is delicious. The sweet peach tastes incredible with the mozarella and pesto – such a perfect combinaton of flavours. I think you'll enjoy this recipe more than once.

SERVES 4

4 small or 2 large peaches, pits removed, each cut into 8 wedges

80g rocket

400g cherry tomatoes, quartered

125g ball of low-fat mozzarella, torn

Croutons

4 slices of crusty bread, preferably wholemeal

1 tbsp extra-virgin olive oil

pinch of salt

Dressing

4 tbsp green basil pesto

2 tbsp extra-virgin olive oil

juice of 1 lemon

pinch of salt

1 garlic clove, crushed

1 Preheat the oven to 220°C/200°C fan.

2 Start with the croutons. Tear the bread into bite-sized chunks and arrange over a baking tray. Drizzle with the oil and a pinch of salt. Bake for 12–15 minutes, or until golden and crisp.

3 In a large bowl, mix together all the dressing ingredients.

4 Tip the toasted croutons into the bowl with the dressing and add the sliced peaches, rocket, tomatoes and mozzarella. Toss together until everything is coated and serve.

FEEL GOOD FACT

Peaches are a good source of vitamin C, as are cherry tomatoes.

SMALL BUT SATISFYING

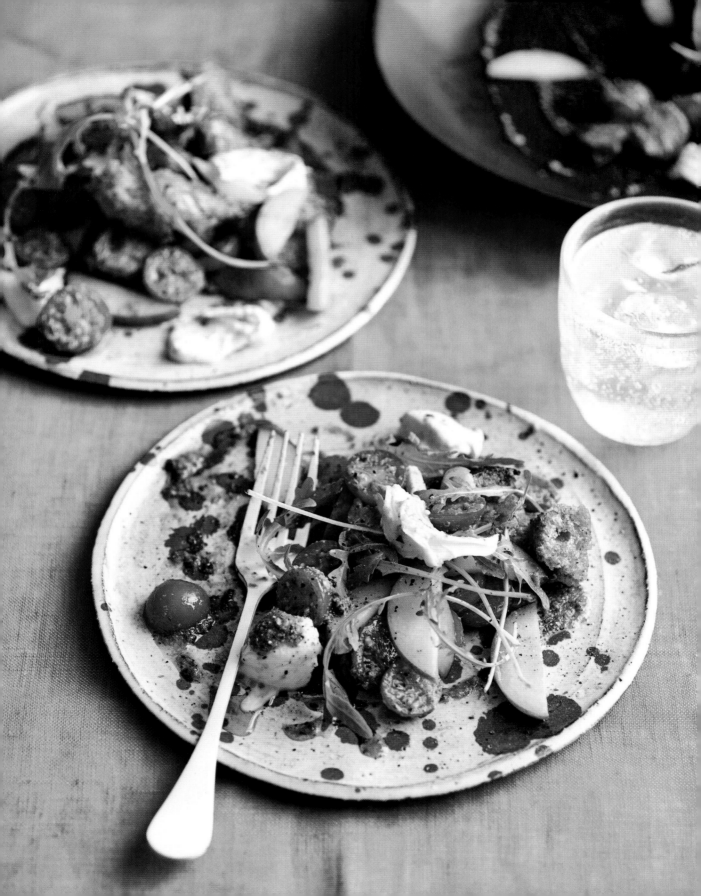

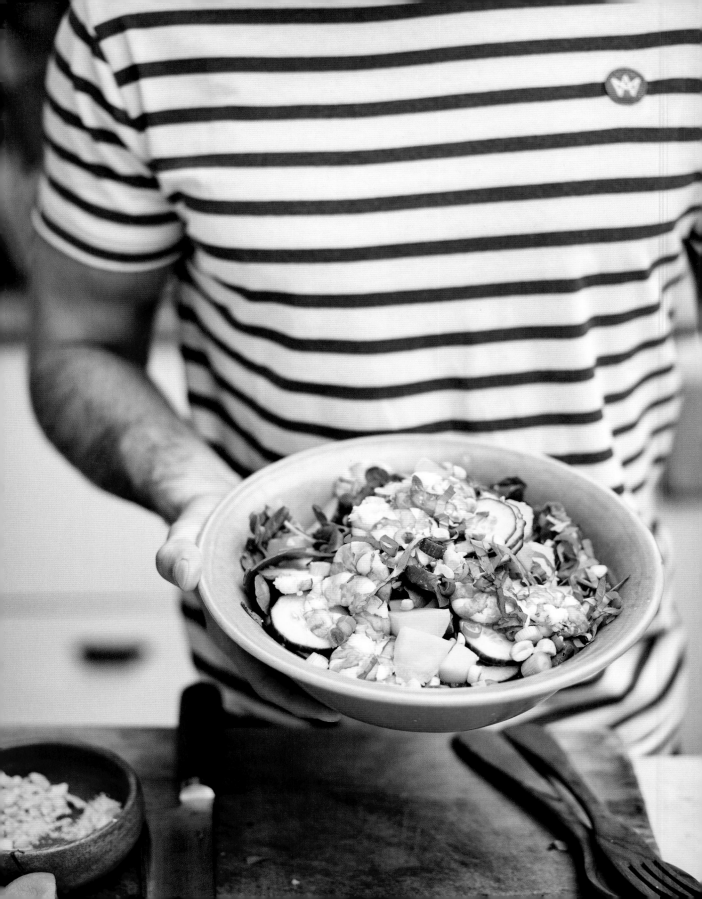

PRAWN, MANGO & CUCUMBER SALAD

I love adding fresh fruit to salads. It takes them to another level and makes them feel so fresh and summery, even if the sun isn't shining. This one is so simple and easy to throw together, but looks very impressive. Give this a go next time your friends come over for a BBQ.

SERVES 4

300g cooked, peeled prawns
  (frozen and defrosted or chilled)

1 large ripe mango, peeled, flesh cubed

4 spring onions, thinly sliced

80g watercress

½ cucumber, thinly sliced into rounds

10g (small handful of) fresh basil

10g (small handful of) fresh coriander

2 tbsp cashews or peanuts,
  roughly chopped

Dressing

2 tbsp lime juice

1 tsp maple syrup

1 tsp sesame oil

¼–½ tsp chilli flakes

1 tsp fish sauce or light soy sauce

1 Combine the dressing ingredients in a mixing bowl.

2 Add the prawns, mango cubes, spring onions, watercress and cucumber. Mix together.

3 Tip the salad into a serving bowl and garnish with the chopped herbs and nuts.

JOE'S TIPS

- Use half a pineapple, diced into small cubes, or 2 Pink Lady apples, diced, in place of the mango.
- Try pea shoots or mixed salad leaves in place of the watercress.
- Switch the coriander or basil for fresh mint.
- To make it more substantial, double the dressing ingredients and mix in 80g cooked rice vermicelli (cook them by soaking in a bowl of boiling water for 4 minutes, then drain and rinse under cold water).

FEEL GOOD FACT

Prawns are an excellent low-fat source of protein, and are also rich in vitamins B12 and E, while mango helps promote healthy digestion and is a good source of vitamins A and C.

BEETROOT, ORANGE & CUMIN SALAD

Beetroot is an amazing vegetable that contains so many fantastic nutrients for the body. This is a recipe that brings a few unusual flavours together and for some reason it just works so well. It's light and fresh and one that you'll definitely polish off!

SERVES 4

1 tsp sesame seeds

1 tsp cumin seeds

1 tsp coriander seeds

1 tbsp olive oil

250g pack of pre-cooked beetroot (not in vinegar), drained and sliced

finely grated zest and juice of 1 orange

4 tbsp low-fat Greek yoghurt

1 small garlic clove, crushed

2 sprigs of fresh mint, leaves picked and roughly chopped

salt

1 Toast the sesame, cumin and coriander seeds in a medium, dry frying pan over a medium heat until fragrant. Remove from the pan to a pestle and mortar and bash a few times to break up the seeds a bit. Set aside.

2 Place the pan back on the heat, add the olive oil, then add the sliced beets and cook on both sides until the colour has changed to a slightly pinker hue, about 5 minutes.

3 Add the orange zest and juice to the pan with a pinch of salt and cook, stirring occasionally, until the juice has reduced down to a tablespoon or so.

4 Mix the yoghurt with the garlic and a pinch of salt, then spread over a plate in a circle shape. Top with the cooked beets and the juices from the pan, then sprinkle with the crushed seeds and the chopped mint.

FEEL GOOD FACT

Beetroot are good for reducing blood pressure and improving exercise endurance by increasing the flow of oxygen in the bloodstream to the muscles. Orange, rich in vitamin C, provides a natural sweetness that counters the earthiness of the beetroot.

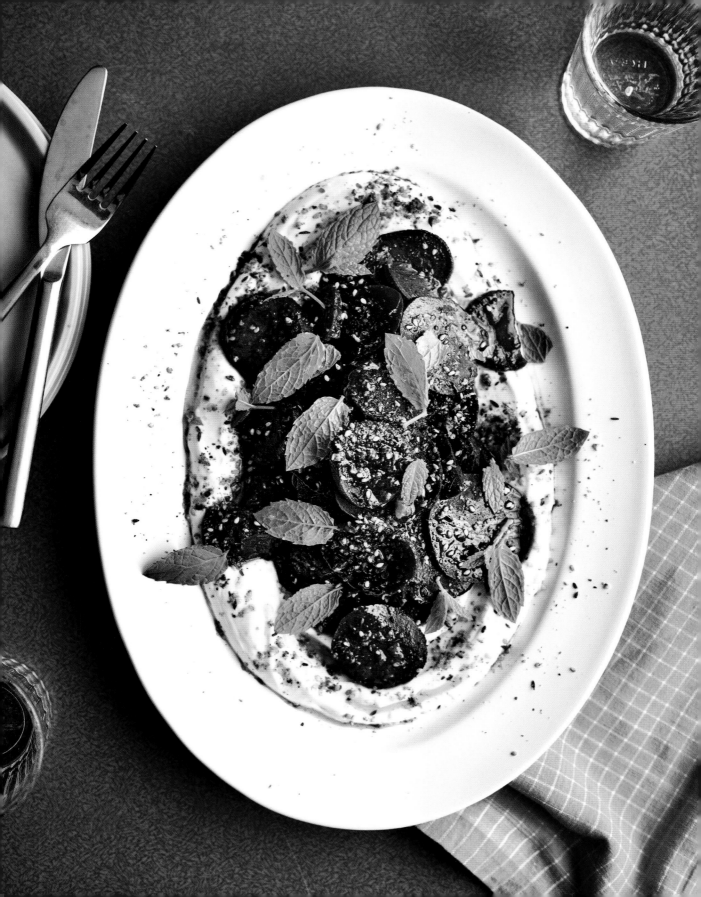

LENTIL SALAD WITH YOGHURT, SUN-DRIED TOMATOES & BASIL

Lentils are a such brilliant source of fibre and protein and something I try to eat at least once a week. The flavours of this salad get better when they marinate for a bit, so this is perfect to make in the evening for the next day's lunchbox.

SERVES 4

120g low-fat natural yoghurt

1 garlic clove, crushed

1 tbsp extra-virgin olive oil

1 tbsp balsamic vinegar

juice of ½ lemon

1 tsp Dijon mustard

75g sun-dried tomatoes (packed in oil), drained

250g pouch of cooked beluga or Puy lentils or 400-g tin of lentils, drained and rinsed

80g rocket

50g walnuts, roughly chopped

50g feta cheese, crumbled

10g (small handful of) fresh basil leaves, torn

salt

1 In a medium bowl, mix together the yoghurt, garlic, olive oil, balsamic vinegar, lemon juice and mustard.

2 Roughly chop the sun-dried tomatoes and stir into the yoghurt mixture along with the cooked lentils. Taste and season with salt, as needed, then gently fold in the rocket.

3 Tip out onto a serving plate and top with the walnuts, feta and fresh basil.

JOE'S TIP

Using yoghurt to dress a salad is an easy, healthy option for when you want that creamy texture, but a lower-fat meal.

SMALL BUT SATISFYING

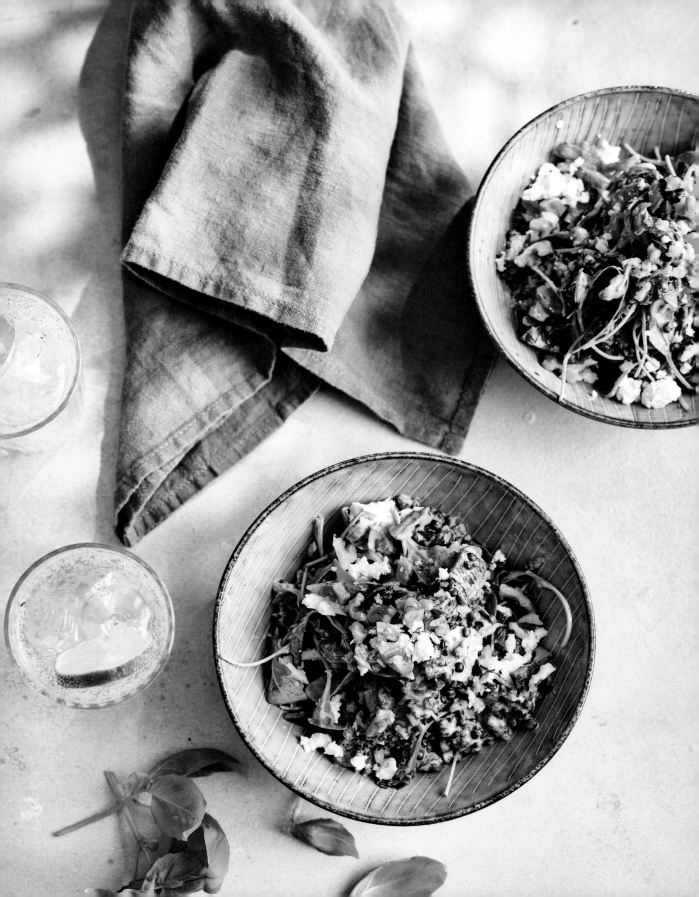

ROASTED CARROTS & BUTTER BEANS WITH HERBY YOGHURT DRESSING

Roasting carrots boosts their natural sweetness and makes them taste so delicious. Combined with the butter beans, this is a really filling salad, guaranteed to keep you feeling satisfied until your next meal.

SERVES 4

400g carrots

1 tbsp olive oil

2 tsp cumin seeds

pinch of salt

400g tin of butter beans, drained but not rinsed

40g pumpkin seeds

Dressing

4 tbsp natural yoghurt

handful of fresh coriander leaves, plus extra to serve

handful of fresh flat-leaf parsley leaves, plus extra to serve

1 garlic clove, crushed

juice of ½ lemon

pinch of salt

1 Preheat the oven to 200°C/180°C fan.

2 Peel the carrots and, if they have leafy tops, trim them. Cut any fat carrots in half or into quarters down their lengths. Place on a baking tray, drizzle with half of the olive oil, sprinkle with the cumin seeds and a pinch of salt, then toss together.

3 Roast the carrots in the oven for 25 minutes.

4 Remove the tray from the oven, add the drained beans, the remaining oil and the pumpkin seeds to the tray. Return to the oven for a further 20–25 minutes until the carrots are starting to caramelise and the beans are crispy and some have popped.

5 Blitz all of the dressing ingredients together with a hand blender (or in a free-standing blender) until smooth.

6 Dish the contents of the tray up onto a serving plate. Pour the dressing over and garnish with more fresh herbs, to serve.

FEEL GOOD FACT

Eating carrots with a source of fat (such as the oil used to roast them and the yoghurt in the dressing) helps the body absorb the vitamin A they contain. Vitamin A is important for eye health, skin health and immune function.

JOE'S TIP

The herby yoghurt dressing is really versatile, so keep any leftovers to enjoy with some grilled chicken or fish the next day.

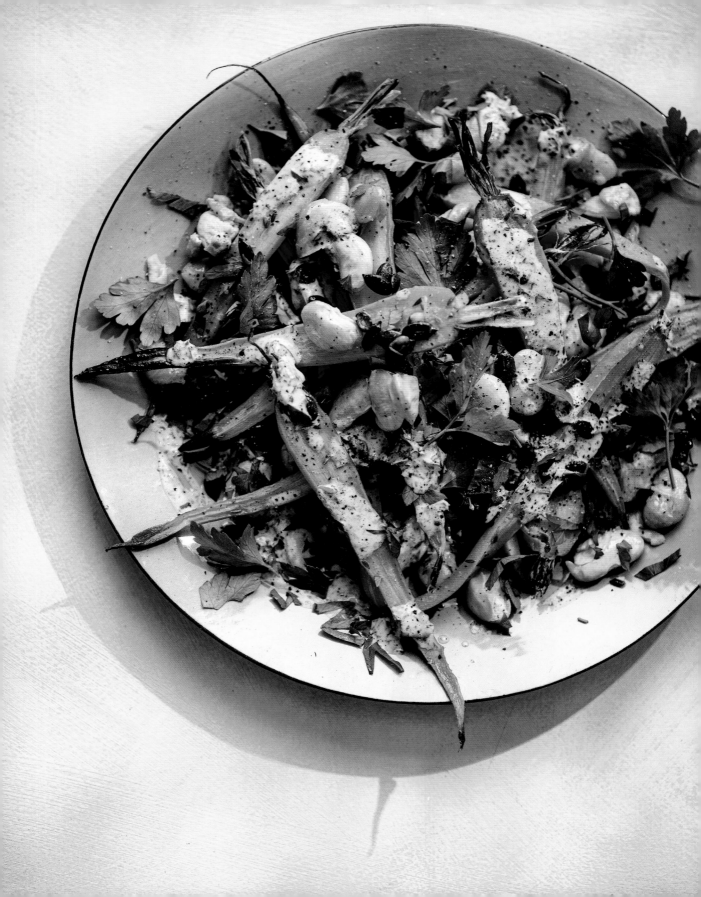

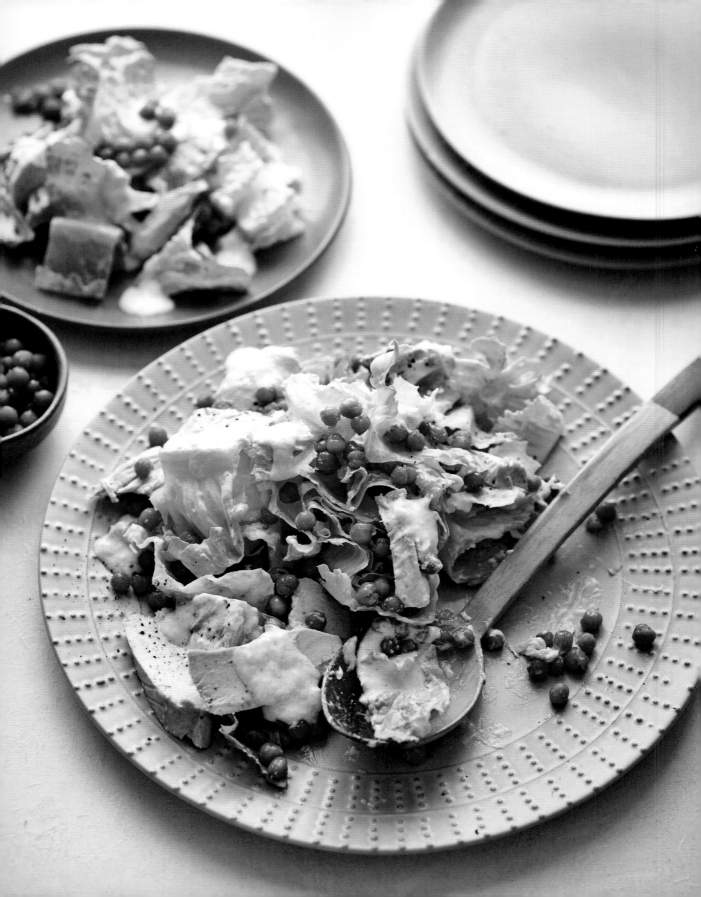

CHICKEN CAESAR SALAD WITH CRISPY CHICKPEA CROUTONS

This is a proper Wicksy special – a healthy spin on an old favourite. I use roasted chickpeas – the high-protein heroes – instead of fried bread croutons and yoghurt instead of mayo in the dressing. It's a really nice swap and tastes wonderful.

SERVES 4

400g tin of chickpeas, drained but not rinsed

1 tbsp light olive oil

½ tsp garlic granules

pinch of salt

2 heads of romaine lettuce

2 cooked skinless chicken breasts, shredded

Dressing

75g 0%-fat Greek yoghurt

1 tbsp lemon juice

1 tbsp extra-virgin olive oil

½ tsp Worcestershire sauce (see Tip)

½ tsp Dijon mustard

10g Parmesan cheese, grated

1 garlic clove, crushed

¼ tsp honey

grated zest of ¼ lemon

1 Preheat the oven to 200°C/180°C fan.

2 Combine all of the dressing ingredients in a small bowl and set aside.

3 Tip the chickpeas onto a rimmed baking tray and drizzle with the olive oil. Sprinkle with the garlic granules and salt, then shake the tray to coat the chickpeas. Bake for 25–30 minutes until crisp.

4 Wash and dry the romaine lettuce, chop it into 3cm chunks and place in a large bowl. Add the shredded chicken and the dressing and toss together to coat. Top with the crunchy chickpeas and serve.

JOE'S TIP

You can use 3 anchovy fillets, mashed with the back of a fork into a paste, instead of the Worcestershire sauce, if you like.

SMALL BUT SATISFYING

ASPARAGUS, BULGUR & EGG SALAD WITH MISO DRESSING

This is a belter of a recipe – a genuine feel good meal. Bulgur wheat is an amazing energy source and the miso paste is packed with minerals and vitamins. Miso is also a fermented food, which provides the gut with beneficial bacteria that helps us stay healthy and happy. It's an all-round winner.

SERVES 4

150g bulgur wheat
½ low-salt vegetable stock cube
500g asparagus
4 large eggs
handful of watercress
handful of fresh basil
freshly ground black pepper

Miso Dressing

3 tbsp extra-virgin olive oil
1 tbsp lemon juice
2 tbsp white or brown miso paste
1 tbsp water
1 garlic clove, crushed

1 Put the bulgur wheat in a small saucepan, cover with 230ml water and crumble in the stock cube. Bring to the boil over a high heat, then stir, reduce to a simmer and cook, covered with a lid, for 10 minutes.

2 Remove the pan from the heat and leave to steam, still covered with the lid, for 5 minutes.

3 Snap off the tough ends of the asparagus and discard. Cut the stalks of asparagus in half lengthways if they are large. Bring a medium pan of water to the boil and add the asparagus stalks, cook for 2 minutes, then remove with tongs to a plate.

4 Reduce the heat under the pan to bring the water to a simmer. Gently lower in the eggs and cook for 5½ minutes, then drain and pop into a bowl of cold water.

5 When cool enough to handle, peel the soft-boiled eggs and cut in half.

6 Shake the dressing ingredients together in a small, lidded jar.

7 To serve, divide the bulgur between bowls, drizzle on the dressing and top each with a halved egg and some of the asparagus and watercress. Finish with a sprinkling of freshly torn basil and a grinding of black pepper.

SMALL BUT SATISFYING

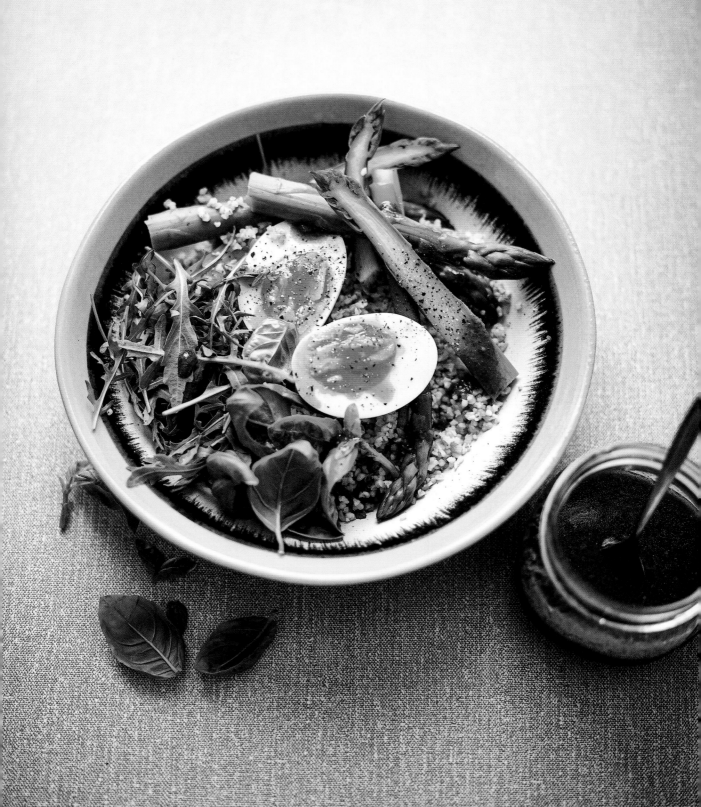

THAI-STYLE SWEET POTATO & SUGAR SNAP SALAD

This Thai-inspired salad is a real winner – packed with so much flavour. It's good on its own as a light lunch, but I also think it makes a great side. Try serving it alongside one of the other Thai-style curries in this book (the Peanut Butter and Coconut Vegetable Curry on page 230 or the Thai Green Chicken and Pea Curry on page 144) for a proper feast.

SERVES 4

600g sweet potatoes, peeled and cut into 2cm thick wedges

1 tbsp light olive oil

pinch of salt

100g sugar snap peas

2 spring onions, thinly sliced

handful of salted peanuts, roughly chopped

Coconut and Coriander Dressing

80g dairy-free coconut yoghurt or coconut milk

20g (big handful of) fresh coriander, roughly chopped

1 green chilli, seeds removed, roughly chopped

1 tbsp fresh ginger, grated

2 tbsp soy sauce

1 tsp runny honey or maple syrup

juice of 1 lime

1 garlic clove, crushed

1 Preheat the oven to 200°C/180°C fan.

2 Place the sweet potato wedges on a baking tray, drizzle with the oil and a pinch of salt, toss together and spread out into an even layer. Bake for 30–40 minutes, flipping halfway through, until golden and soft.

3 Blitz together all of the dressing ingredients using a hand or free-standing blender.

4 Transfer the warm sweet potato wedges to a plate and scatter over the sugar snap peas. Pour over the dressing and scatter on the spring onions and peanuts.

SMALL BUT SATISFYING

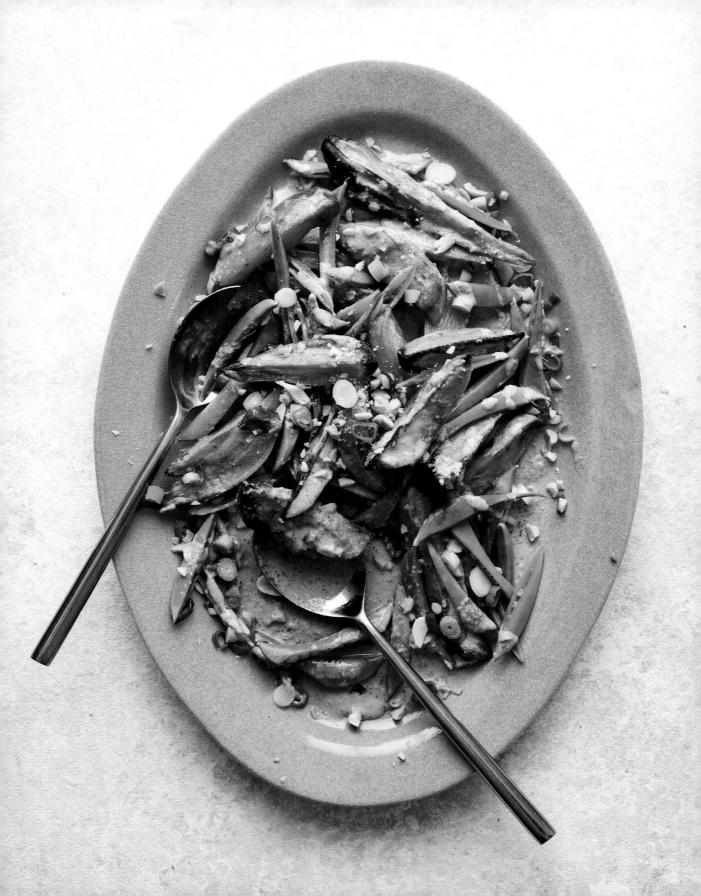

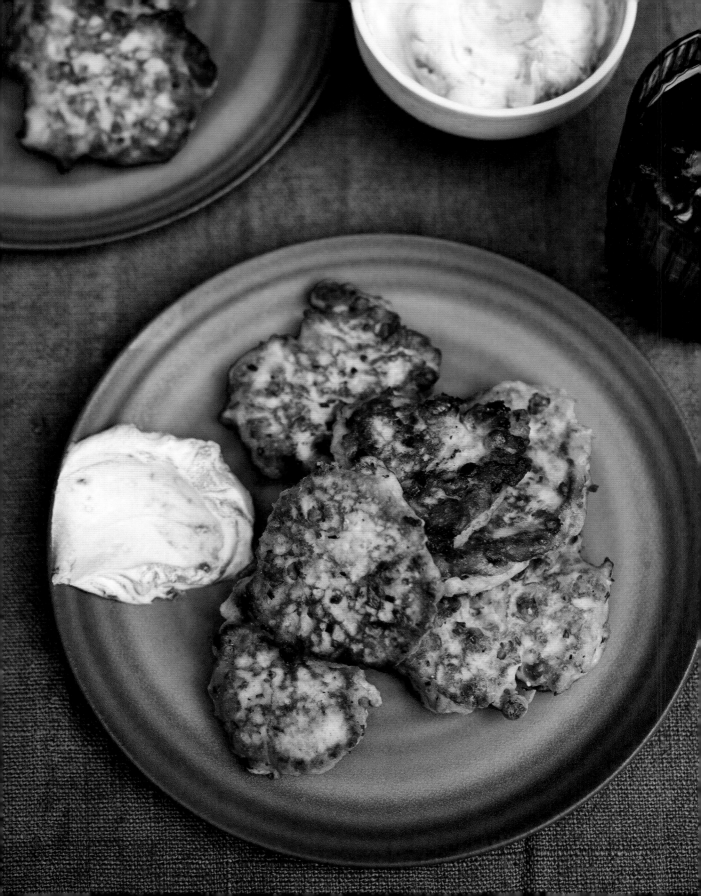

PEA & RICOTTA FRITTERS WITH HARISSA YOGHURT

If you haven't tasted harissa before, this recipe is just for you. It's such a special flavour and really works well when mixed in with the yoghurt as a dip. Fritters are another great way of getting more veg into your diet, too. They're super easy to make with frozen peas, which are just as healthy and nutritious as fresh ones.

SERVES 4

200g frozen peas

250g ricotta cheese

10g (small handful) chives, finely chopped

10g (small handful) fresh mint leaves, finely chopped

4 eggs

15g vegetarian hard cheese or Parmesan, finely grated

40g fresh or dried breadcrumbs

3 tbsp plain white or wholemeal flour

2–3 tbsp light olive oil, for frying

1 tbsp harissa

4 tbsp natural yoghurt

1 Defrost the peas by placing them in a bowl and covering with boiling water. Leave to stand for a few minutes, then drain well and set aside.

2 In a medium bowl, mix together the ricotta, chives, mint leaves, eggs, grated cheese, breadcrumbs and flour. Tip in the drained peas and stir through.

3 Heat a frying pan over a medium heat with enough olive oil to thinly coat the base of the pan. Add a heaped teaspoonful of the fritter mixture and spread out a little with the back of your spoon. Fry until golden underneath, then flip with a metal spatula – the fritters can be delicate if you try to flip them too early, so do make sure they're properly cooked underneath before you flip.

4 Repeat with the remaining batter, removing the fritters to a plate as they're ready.

5 Swirl the harissa through the yoghurt in a small bowl and serve alongside the warm fritters.

JOE'S TIPS

- For a brunch classic, turn these into corn fritters. Replace the frozen peas with frozen sweetcorn and replace the mint with fresh coriander. They go great with some smashed avocado and an egg!
- If the harissa is too spicy for the kids, instead mix ½ tsp smoked paprika and 1 small crushed garlic clove into the yoghurt with a pinch of salt.
- As a simple lunch, serve the fritters with a mixed salad.

SPINACH & FETA BALL WRAPS WITH BEETROOT HUMMUS

Life is so much better with cheesy stuff in it, don't you think? These spinach and feta cheese balls taste unreal with beetroot hummus on a nice, warm, wholemeal wrap. If you want a healthy lunch on the go, wrap it tightly in some foil and enjoy it later in the day.

SERVES 4

Spinach and Feta Balls

1kg frozen chopped spinach, defrosted

150g panko breadcrumbs

2 tsp ground cumin

1 tsp ground coriander

2 medium onions, finely diced

2 tsp garlic granules or 2 garlic cloves, finely grated

6 eggs

4 tbsp extra-virgin olive oil

250g feta cheese

Beetroot Hummus

2 vac-packed cooked beetroots (not in vinegar)

400g tin of chickpeas, drained reserving the liquid

3 tbsp extra virgin olive oil

2 garlic cloves, crushed

2 tbsp lemon juice

2 tbsp tahini (optional)

salt, to taste

To Serve

¼ green cabbage, finely sliced

30g fresh coriander, roughly chopped

1 tbsp apple cider vinegar or lemon juice

pinch of salt

8 wholemeal wraps, warmed

lemon wedges

1 Preheat the oven to 200°C/180°C fan and line two baking trays with baking paper.

2 Place the defrosted spinach in a colander in the sink and squeeze to remove most of the water. Put the squeezed spinach into a large bowl and add the remaining spinach ball ingredients apart from the feta. Mix together until everything is distributed evenly (I use my hands here to squish it together). Finally, crumble the feta cheese into the bowl and mix together.

3 Take heaped tablespoons of the mixture, roll into balls and place on the lined baking trays, spacing them about 3cm apart. Bake for 25–30 minutes until golden and slightly crisp.

4 To make the hummus, combine the beetroots, chickpeas, olive oil, garlic, lemon juice and tahini (if using) in a blender or food processor. Add 80ml of the liquid from the tin of chickpeas and blitz until smooth. Add salt to taste and blitz again. You can loosen the mixture by adding more chickpea liquid, if needed.

5 Place the finely sliced cabbage and coriander in a medium bowl and drizzle over the apple cider vinegar or lemon juice and a pinch of salt. Use your hands to scrunch and massage the cabbage to help it break down and soften a bit.

6 Serve the wraps with the spinach and feta balls, beetroot hummus, scrunched cabbage and lemon wedges for squeezing over, and let everyone dig in.

JOE'S TIP

For a shortcut, get a tub of shop-bought hummus and either blitz with a couple of vac-packed beetroot or roughly chop up the beetroot and fold through the hummus.

SMALL BUT SATISFYING

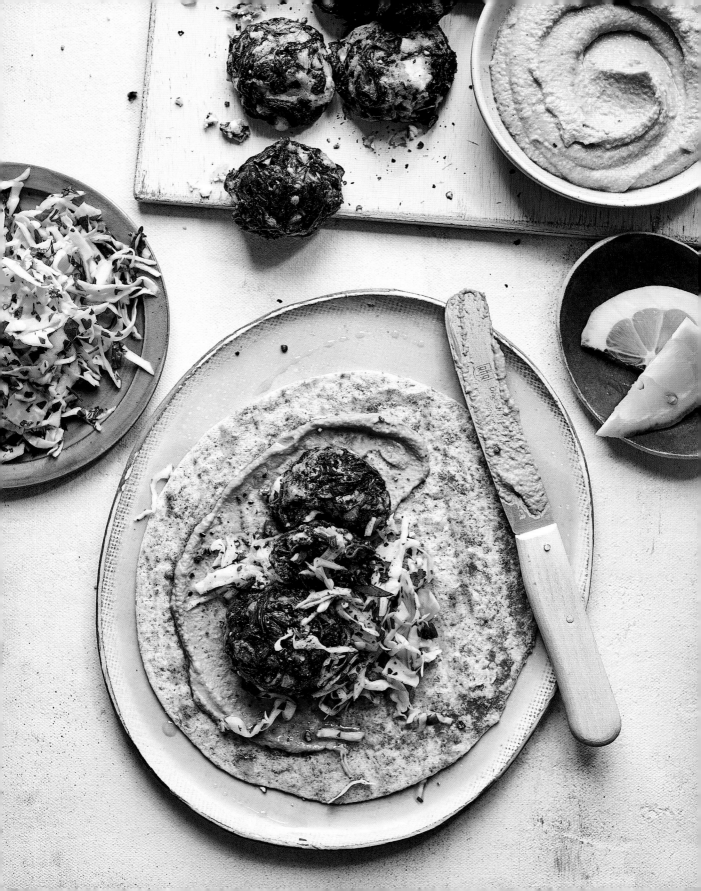

THAI LETTUCE CUPS WITH SPICED TURKEY & RICE

These Thai-style lettuce cups are really fun to build and eat with kids or friends. It's great to lay all the cooked ingredients out on the table and then all get stuck in, building your own sweet, sour, hot and crunchy treats.

SERVES 4

2 tbsp coconut oil

2 banana shallots, thinly sliced

500g minced turkey

4 fresh or frozen lime leaves
  (or 1–2 tbsp green Thai curry paste)

2 courgettes, cut into 1cm cubes

1 red chilli, seeds removed, finely chopped

handful of fresh coriander,
  roughly chopped

handful of fresh mint leaves,
  roughly chopped

handful of Thai basil (or regular basil),
  roughly chopped

180g jasmine rice

300ml water

2 romaine lettuce hearts, leaves separated
  and rinsed

1 carrot, julienned or peeled into ribbons
  with a vegetable peeler

salt

Dressing

50ml lime juice

2 tbsp maple syrup

1 garlic clove, crushed

1 tbsp fish sauce

2 tsp water

1 Heat 1 tablespoon of the coconut oil in a large, non-stick frying pan over a medium-low heat. Once melted, add the shallots and cook for 7–10 minutes until they start to turn golden. Add the turkey mince, breaking it up with your spoon, and cook until any liquid that it releases has cooked off. Stir in the lime leaves (or curry paste, if using) and cook for 1 minute. Tip into a bowl.

2 Wipe out the pan with kitchen paper and return it to the heat. Add the remaining coconut oil and, once melted, add the diced courgette with a pinch of salt. Cook over a medium heat until golden, then stir the turkey mince mixture back in along with the chilli. Remove from the heat and set aside.

3 Mix all of the dressing ingredients together and stir into the turkey mixture along with the chopped herbs.

4 Wash the rice until the water runs mostly clear, then tip into a medium saucepan and add the water and a pinch of salt. Bring to the boil over a high heat, then reduce the heat to low, cover the pan with a lid and cook for 10 minutes. Remove from the heat and leave the lid on for a further 7 minutes to steam.

5 To serve, fill each lettuce leaf with some of the jasmine rice, the turkey mixture and julienned carrot.

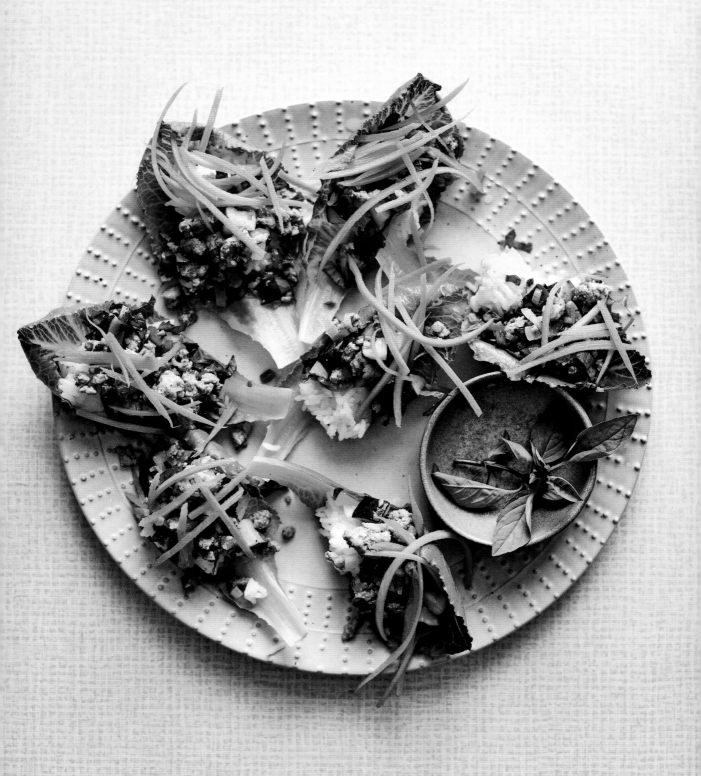

SPICED YOGHURT-COATED CARROT & PANEER WRAPS WITH BROCCOLI SLAW

These gorgeous, colourful wraps are awesome and super healthy. The spices give them lots of flavour and they go so well with the sweet roasted carrots. They will make a perfect lunch at home or can be wrapped in foil and eaten on the go.

SERVES 4

200g 0%-fat Greek yoghurt

¼ tsp ground turmeric

2 tsp ground coriander

1 tsp garam masala

½ tsp chilli powder

2 tsp cumin seeds

¼ tsp salt

1 tbsp grated fresh ginger

3 garlic cloves, crushed

juice of ½ lemon

250g paneer cheese, cut into 2cm cubes

750g carrots, cut into 2cm chunks

1 tbsp coconut oil

8 wholemeal tortillas

handful of fresh coriander, roughly chopped

Broccoli Slaw

1 small head of broccoli

1 red onion, finely chopped

30g raisins

50g 0%-fat Greek yoghurt

1 tbsp low-fat mayonnaise

juice of 1 lemon

pinch of salt

1 In a large bowl, mix the yoghurt, spices, salt, ginger, garlic and lemon juice into a smooth paste. Add the paneer cubes and carrot chunks and toss together until thoroughly coated. Set aside for 15 minutes.

2 Preheat the oven to 200°C/180°C fan.

3 Scoop the coconut oil onto a large, rimmed baking tray and place in the oven for 1 minute, or until the oil has melted. Tilt the tray to spread the oil over the surface, then add the contents of the bowl and spread out into an even layer. Bake for 40–50 minutes, flipping the carrots and paneer over after 30 minutes, until the carrots are soft and the paneer is starting to caramelise.

4 Meanwhile, make the slaw. Cut the thick stem off the base of the broccoli, cut away the outer tough layer and then thinly slice the tender part of the stem into matchsticks. Cut the head of the broccoli thinly, starting at the flowery top and working towards the stem. Add all of this to a medium bowl along with the onion, raisins, yoghurt, mayo, lemon juice and salt. Mix together until completely coated and combined.

5 Warm the tortillas according to the packet instructions.

6 Serve the warmed tortillas topped with the warm paneer mixture and the slaw, scattered with coriander. Fold or roll as you like.

SMALL BUT SATISFYING

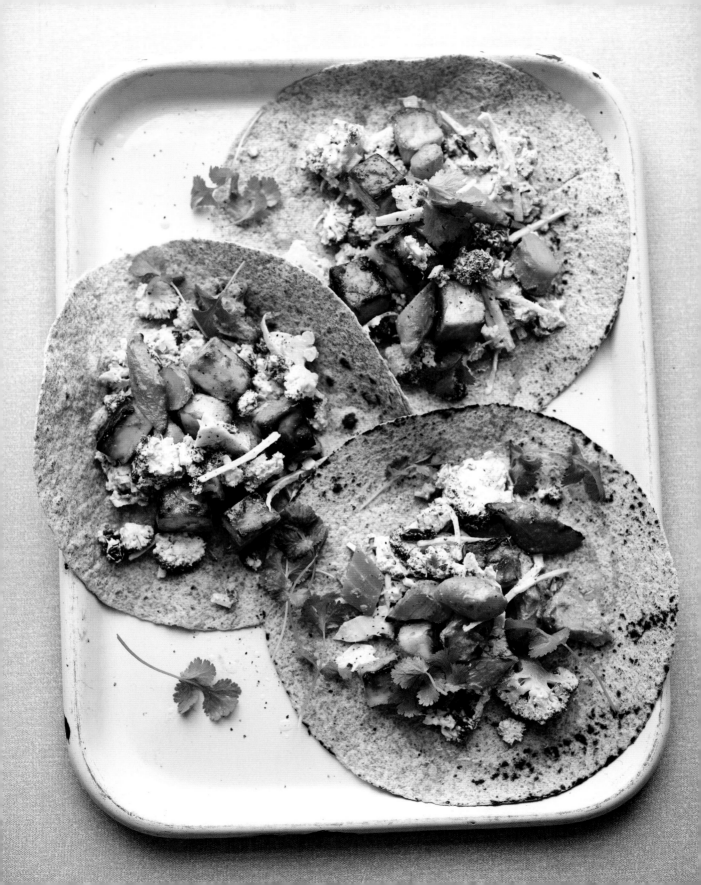

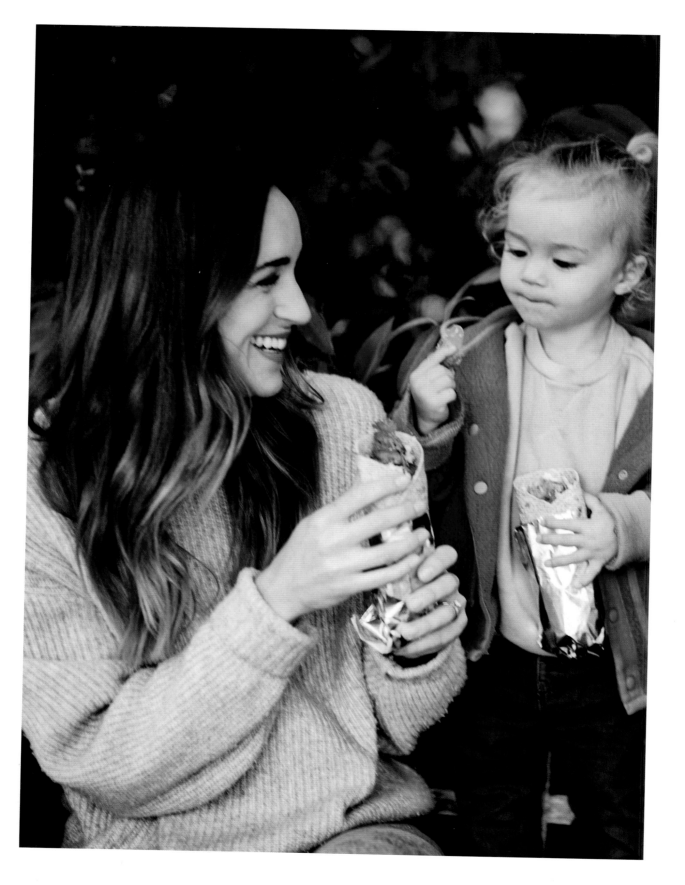

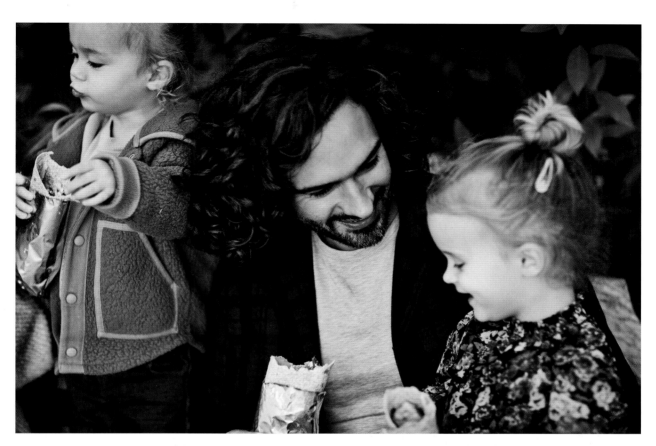

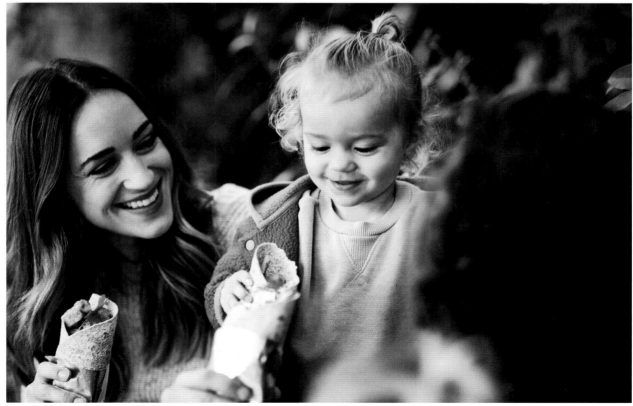

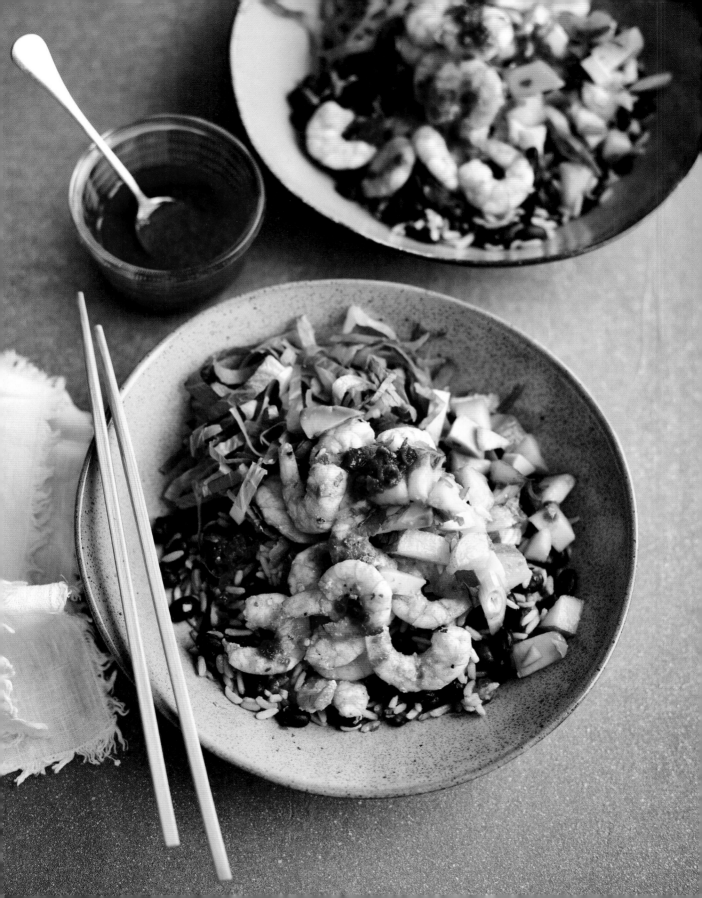

HARISSA PRAWN BOWLS WITH PEACH SALSA

Unbelievable flavours in this colourful dish. Harissa is one of my favourite things to cook with. It's hard to describe how it tastes, but I promise it's spicy and delicious. You can find little jars of harissa in the herb and spice section in the supermarket.

SERVES 4

Peach Salsa

3 medium, ripe peaches

1 avocado

finely grated zest and juice of ½ lime

handful of fresh coriander, roughly chopped

2 spring onions, thinly sliced

pinch of salt

Spiced Prawns

1 tbsp light olive oil

360g frozen raw king prawns

½ tsp smoked paprika

½ tsp garlic granules

½ tsp dried oregano

pinch of cayenne pepper

pinch of freshly ground black pepper

Dressing

1 tbsp harissa

3 tbsp extra-virgin olive oil

2 tbsp lime juice

½ tsp runny honey

To Serve

300g cooked brown rice

400g tin of black beans, drained and rinsed

2 heads of gem lettuce, shredded

1 First, make the peach salsa. Remove the peach stones then dice the flesh finely. Cut the avocado in half and remove the stone, then scoop out the flesh and roughly dice. Add the peach and avocado to a medium bowl with the remaining salsa ingredients, stir and set aside.

2 For the spiced prawns, heat the light olive oil in a large frying pan over a high heat. Add the frozen prawns and cook until fully defrosted and pink. Stir in the smoked paprika, garlic, oregano, cayenne and black pepper. When the prawns are fully coated, remove from the heat and set aside.

3 Mix together all the dressing ingredients in a small bowl or jar.

4 Combine the cooked brown rice and black beans, then divide between 4 bowls. Top with the shredded lettuce, the cooked prawns and the salsa. Drizzle with the dressing and serve.

FEEL GOOD FACT

With low-fat, high-protein prawns, high-fibre black beans, monounsaturated fats from the avocado and healthy carbs from the brown rice, this has everything you need for a well-balanced meal.

PHO-INSPIRED COD & RICE NOODLE SOUP

Pho is a really flavourful Vietnamese soup broth that is full of delicious spices and aromas. The smell of this cooking will really get your tastebuds going! It's easy to buy pre-portioned boneless, skinless cod fillets, so prep time is quite minimal. Enjoy!

SERVES 4

2 star anise

10cm cinnamon stick

30g fresh ginger

1 onion, peeled and quartered

1 apple, cored, cut into eighths

1 medium carrot, cut into 3cm chunks

2 chicken stock cubes

2 litres water

1 tsp coriander seeds

1 tsp black peppercorns

2 tsp runny honey

2 tbsp fish sauce or soy sauce

2 x 140g fillets of cod, cut into
    3cm chunks

2 pak choi, cut into quarters lengthways

200g rice stick noodles

200g beansprouts

handful of fresh coriander,
    roughly chopped

handful of Thai basil or regular basil,
    roughly chopped

1 small onion, very thinly sliced

To Serve

1 lime, cut into wedges

hoisin sauce

sriracha, or other hot sauce

1 Use metal tongs to toast the star anise, cinnamon stick, whole ginger and onion on the open flame of a gas hob until blackened. If you don't have a gas hob, slice the ginger first, pop into a heavy-based frying pan over a high heat on the stove and toast until the ginger is charred and the spices have darkened.

2 Slice the blackened ginger if you haven't already, then tip the toasted ingredients into a large, heavy-based saucepan along with the apple, carrot, stock cubes, water, coriander seeds, peppercorns and honey. Bring to the boil over a high heat, then reduce to a simmer, cover and cook for 1 hour.

3 Strain out the solids from the broth, then return the broth to the pan. Season with the fish or soy sauce, bring to a simmer, then add the cod and pak choi. Cook for 6–8 minutes until the fish flakes apart easily and the pak choi is tender.

4 Prepare the rice noodles by placing them in a heatproof bowl and covering with boiling water. Leave to stand for 3–5 minutes, then drain and rinse under cold water.

5 Divide the noodles between 4 bowls. Ladle the soup over the noodles and garnish with the beansprouts, herbs and sliced onion. Serve with wedges of lime for squeezing, hoisin sauce and sriracha for drizzling.

FEEL GOOD FACT

Pak choi is a good source of vitamin C (for maintaining skin health). Fish is a fantastic low-fat source of protein, phosphorous, niacin and vitamin B12, so do try to regularly include some in your diet.

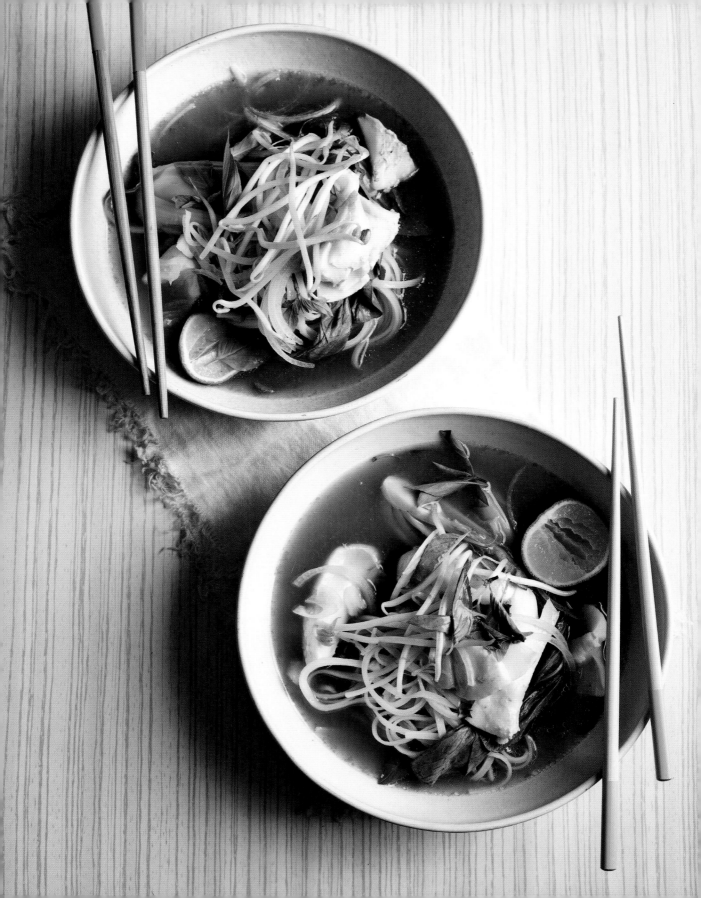

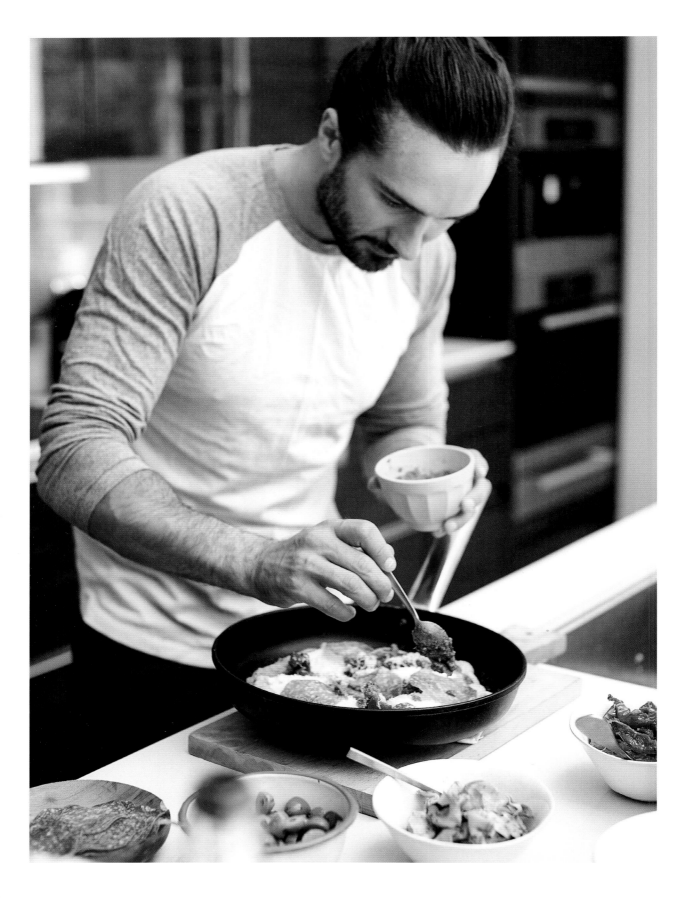

4

COMFORT

favourite fakeaways and
fast-food swaps

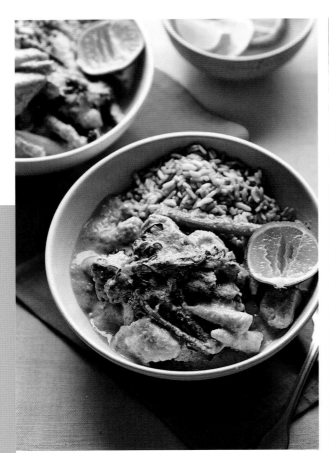

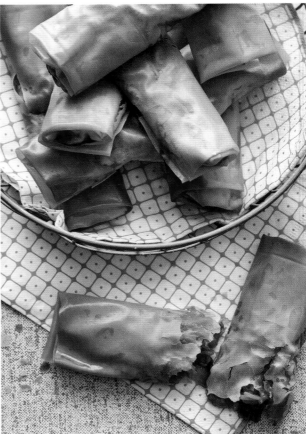

Comfort food, fast food, takeaways… Whatever your particular fix is, there's a healthier version you can swap in with no compromise on flavour. Turn to this chapter whenever you feel the urge to splurge.

There are definitely days we all really fancy a burger or some nachos. I know I do! But when I do over-indulge, I often feel sluggish later that day or even the next day. That's why I love to have these recipes up my sleeve. They have all the comfort and all of the flavour, but less of the bad stuff. Perfect!

The frying pan pizza on pages 148–150 is a real game-changer for me. Prepping the super-quick dough in advance, knowing it's there ready for when you get in from work or a workout, is just so brilliant. And the kids absolutely love choosing their favourite toppings to add at the end – loads of fun.

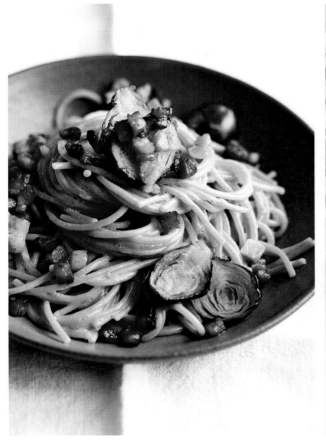

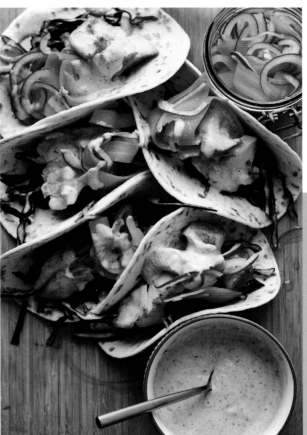

And then there are the burgers. Oh yes.... the burgers! The Chicken Caprese Burger on page 135, with mozarella and pesto, has got to be one of my best creations yet. The Beef and Black Bean Burger on page 132 gives it a good run for its money though – it tastes bangin'.

I also love a good Thai curry, and the Thai Green Chicken and Pea Curry on page 144 ticks all my boxes. It's easy to throw together, big on flavours and it's super healthy, too, with loads of veg.

And for those days when you're feeding a crowd, the two tasty taco recipes on pages 152 and 155 are just perfect for some DIY fun. Bung all the bits down on the table in loads of bowls and everyone can dig in, helping themselves.

SWEET POTATO NACHOS

I mean, come on, look at the photo. How good do they look? Nacho life for the win. This is actually a really healthy recipe with loads of good stuff. It's one of the best things to make as a family and to dive into when it comes out of the oven. Cheese all dripping down your chin… Mess everywhere… Fighting over the last crispy bits!

SERVES 4

4 medium sweet potatoes (around 600g), peeled and sliced into 5mm thick coins

1 tbsp light olive oil

1 tsp salt

60g Cheddar cheese, grated

4 tbsp low-fat natural yoghurt, to serve

Spiced Mince

1 tbsp oil

1 red onion, diced

100g veggie mince or minced beef

½ tsp ground cumin

½ tsp ground coriander

½ tsp smoked paprika

pinch of chilli powder

130g frozen sliced peppers (or the same amount of fresh, sliced)

Refried Beans

400g tin of black beans, drained but liquid reserved

pinch of salt

1 tsp ground cumin

Salsa

200g cherry tomatoes, roughly chopped

big handful of fresh coriander, finely chopped

juice of 1 lime

pinch of salt

1 Preheat the oven to 200°C/180°C fan.

2 Toss the sliced sweet potatoes with the oil and salt on a large baking tray, then spread them out into a single layer (you may need a second baking tray). Roast for 30–40 minutes, flipping them over halfway through, until starting to turn golden.

3 For the spiced mince, heat the oil in a large frying pan over a medium-low heat. Add the onion and cook for about 5 minutes until translucent. Add the mince, breaking it up with your spoon, and cook for a few minutes according to the packet instructions, or until the mince is no longer pink if using beef. Stir in the cumin, coriander, paprika, chilli powder and frozen (or fresh) sliced peppers. Stir until the peppers have defrosted and warmed through (about 5 minutes if using fresh, until softened). Tip into a bowl and set aside.

4 For the refried beans, return the same pan to the heat and add the drained beans along with 100ml of the liquid reserved from the tin, the salt and cumin. Mash with a potato masher in the pan, loosening with more bean liquid as needed, to make a creamy, slightly chunky paste. Remove from the heat and set aside.

5 Mix together all of the salsa ingredients in a small bowl and set aside.

6 Once the potato nachos are roasted, top with spoonfuls of the refried beans, followed by a layer of the mince mixture and finally sprinkle over the grated cheese.

7 Return to the oven for 10–15 minutes until the cheese has melted and crisped up in places.

8 Remove from the oven, top with the salsa and some dollops of yoghurt, then serve.

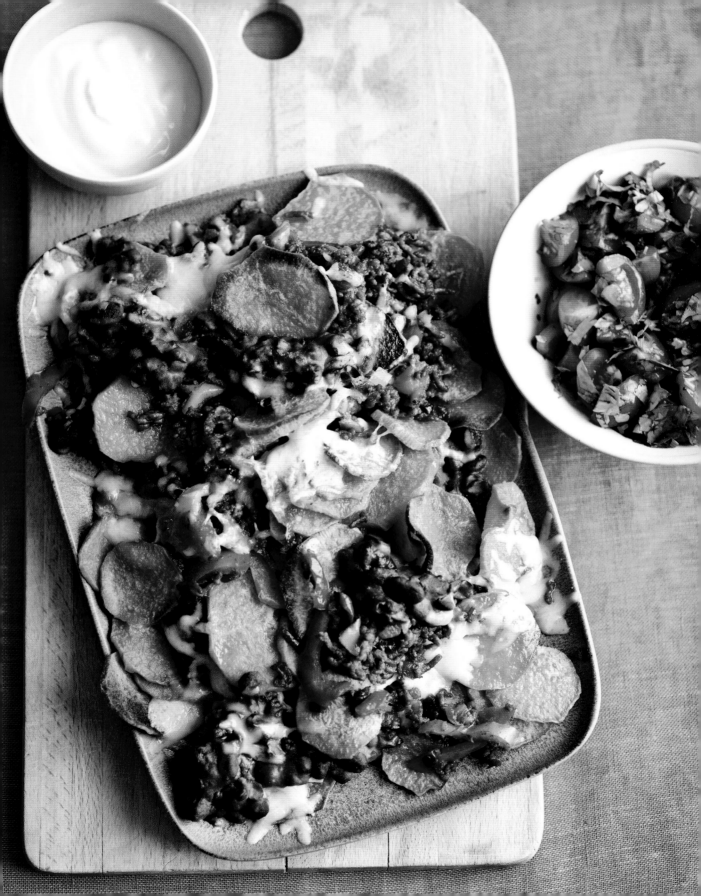

BEEF & BLACK BEAN BURGERS WITH SWEET POTATO SLAW

When it comes to food, nothing makes me happier than a juicy burger. There's nothing more satisfying than a good patty in a bun is there? This combines beef with black beans, so it's high in fibre and protein and tastes bangin'. It goes great with this crunchy Greek yoghurt slaw, too.

MAKES 8 BURGERS / SERVES 4–8 DEPENDING ON HUNGER

400g tin of black beans, drained and rinsed

1 red onion, finely diced

2 tsp smoked paprika

1 tsp ground cumin

300g minced beef (12% fat)

1 large egg

30g panko breadcrumbs

2 tbsp olive oil, for frying

4–8 wholemeal English muffins, halved, to serve

Sweet Potato Slaw

75g 0%-fat Greek yoghurt

1 garlic clove, crushed

2 tbsp apple cider vinegar

1 small sweet potato, peeled and coarsely grated

¼ head of red cabbage, very thinly sliced

1 red onion, finely diced

handful of fresh coriander, roughly chopped

1 Tip the black beans into a large bowl and crush with a potato masher into a chunky paste. Add the onion, smoked paprika and cumin and stir together, then add the beef mince, egg and breadcrumbs and gently incorporate into the mixture until just combined.

2 Divide the mixture into 8 equal balls, then flatten into patties.

3 Heat the oil in a large, non-stick frying pan over a high heat. Cook the patties until browned underneath, 3–5 minutes, then flip and cook on the other side until browned.

4 For the slaw, combine the yoghurt, garlic and vinegar in a medium bowl, then fold in the grated sweet potato, cabbage, onion and coriander.

5 Toast the muffins in a dry pan or on a griddle.

6 Serve the burgers in the toasted muffins, topped with the slaw.

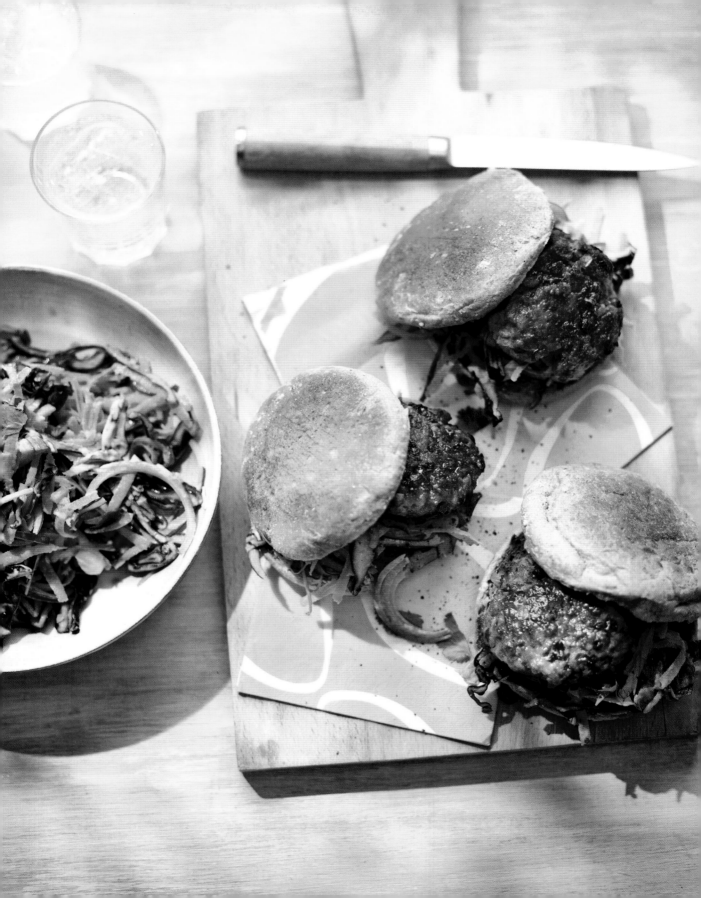

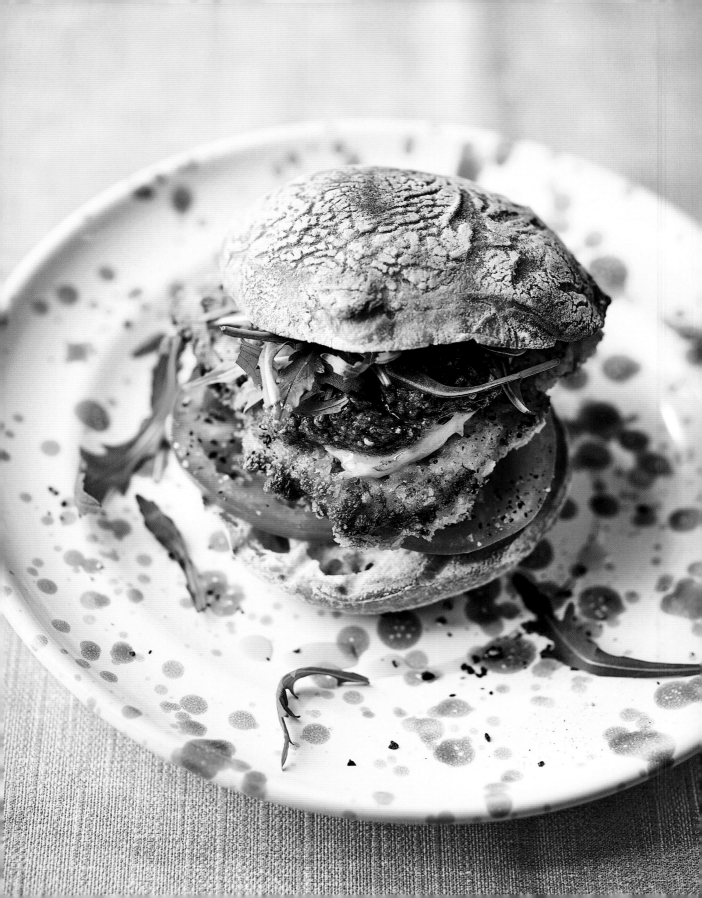

CHICKEN CAPRESE BURGERS

Just look at this burger. Oh my days... It's heavenly, isn't it? I love everything about it. The chicken, mozzarella and pesto are a match made in heaven. Don't skip this recipe because I think it's one of the best burgers I've ever created.

SERVES 4

4 skinless chicken breasts

50g plain flour

1 tsp dried oregano

1 egg

75g panko breadcrumbs

2 tbsp olive oil

salt and freshly ground black pepper

To Serve

1 x 125g ball of mozzarella cheese, drained

4 heaped tsp basil pesto

4 ciabatta rolls, halved

4 medium tomatoes, sliced

handful of fresh rocket

1 Preheat the oven to 220°C/200°C fan and line a large baking tray with baking paper.

2 Take a large piece of baking paper, place a chicken breast on the left half of the paper and fold the right half of the paper over the top. Whack the chicken with the end of a rolling pin until it's an even thickness all over. Set this chicken breast aside and repeat with the remaining chicken. Cut each breast in half so you have 8 smaller pieces in total.

3 Take 3 wide, shallow dishes. In one, mix the flour, dried oregano, a pinch of salt and a pinch of ground black pepper. In the second dish, mix the egg with a pinch of salt. In the third dish, place the panko breadcrumbs. Dip each chicken piece in the flour, the egg and finally the breadcrumbs, shaking off the excess. Place onto the lined baking tray spacing them a few centimetres apart. Drizzle with half of the oil, then flip them all over and drizzle with the remaining oil.

4 Bake for 25–30 minutes, flipping them over halfway through the cooking time, until golden and crisp.

5 Cut the mozzarella into 8 slices and place one slice onto each piece of chicken. Return to the oven for 5 minutes so that the cheese can melt.

6 Remove from the oven and top each piece of chicken with a little pesto. Serve in the ciabatta rolls with the rocket and tomatoes.

JOE'S TIP

I like to serve two pieces of chicken per roll for a larger burger, and one piece of chicken per roll for the kids.

FISH FINGER (OR TOFU) SANDWICHES

Fish finger sandwiches are a classic. If you know, you know. I used to make these all the time with frozen fish fingers, white bread, all doused in Tommy K (ketchup). In this recipe, we are going fresh with easy home-made fish fingers and a healthy tartare or pea sauce. You can use tofu for a veggie version. The tartare sauce is made with yoghurt so you get the creamy flavour with extra protein and the pea sauce is like home-made mushy peas.

SERVES 4

500g white fish, preferably thick fillets, or 450g firm tofu

75g plain white flour

½ tsp smoked paprika

zest of 1 lemon

2 eggs

120g panko breadcrumbs

2 tbsp light olive oil or refined coconut oil

salt and freshly ground black pepper

Pea and Yoghurt Sauce (optional)

100g frozen peas, defrosted and well drained

2 tbsp low-fat Greek yoghurt

1½ tsp lemon juice

1 small garlic clove, crushed

2 tsp finely chopped fresh mint (optional)

pinch of salt

Tartare Sauce (optional)

3 tbsp low-fat Greek yoghurt

2 tbsp lemon juice

4 tbsp finely chopped flat-leaf parsley

1 shallot, finely diced

½ tsp capers, drained and finely chopped

To Serve

4 crusty bread rolls

handful of rocket

1 1 If you are using tofu, press it first. Wrap the block of tofu in a clean tea towel and place on a chopping board, place another chopping board on top and weigh it down with a couple of cookbooks. Leave for 15–30 minutes to drain, then unwrap.

2 Cut the pressed tofu or the fish fillets into 2cm-thick fingers.

3 Get 3 wide, shallow bowls. In one bowl, place the flour with the smoked paprika, lemon zest and a pinch each of salt and freshly ground black pepper, and mix lightly to combine. Crack the eggs into the second bowl and lightly whisk with a pinch of salt. Place the panko breadcrumbs in the third bowl.

4 Dip each finger of tofu or fish into the flour, then into the egg, then into the breadcrumbs until coated. Place the finished fingers onto a tray.

5 Heat the oil in a large frying pan. Add the breadcrumbed fingers and cook until browned underneath, then turn and cook on all sides until golden all over. Remove to a plate.

6 To make the pea and yoghurt sauce, if using, blitz all the ingredients with a hand blender in a jug, or in a free-standing blender, until roughly puréed.

7 To make the tartare sauce, if using, add all the ingredients to a small bowl and stir until combined.

8 Serve the fish or tofu fingers in a halved crusty roll with the sauce of your choice and a handful of rocket leaves.

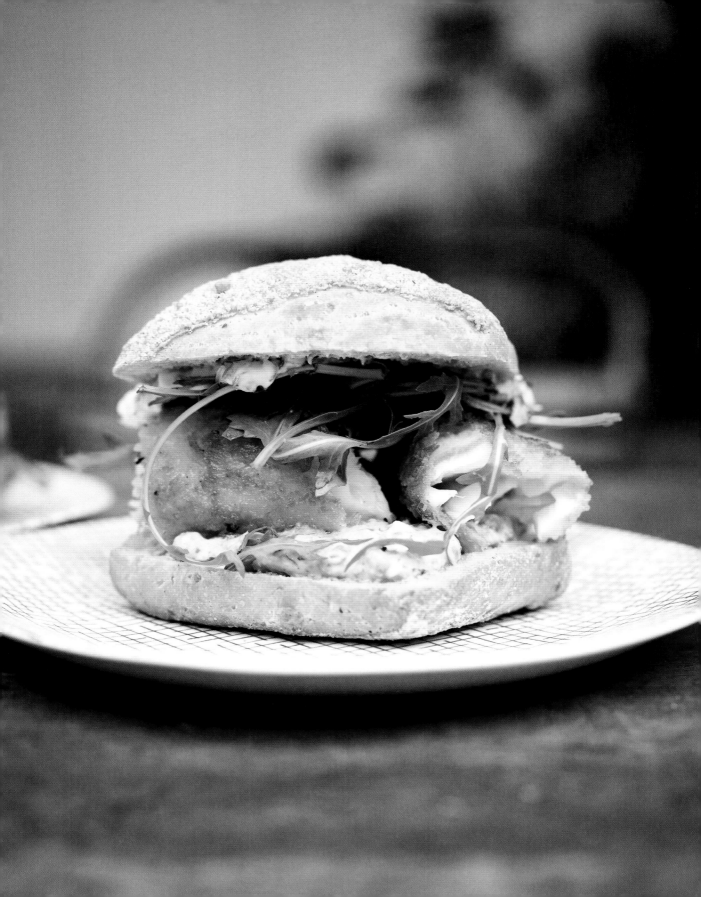

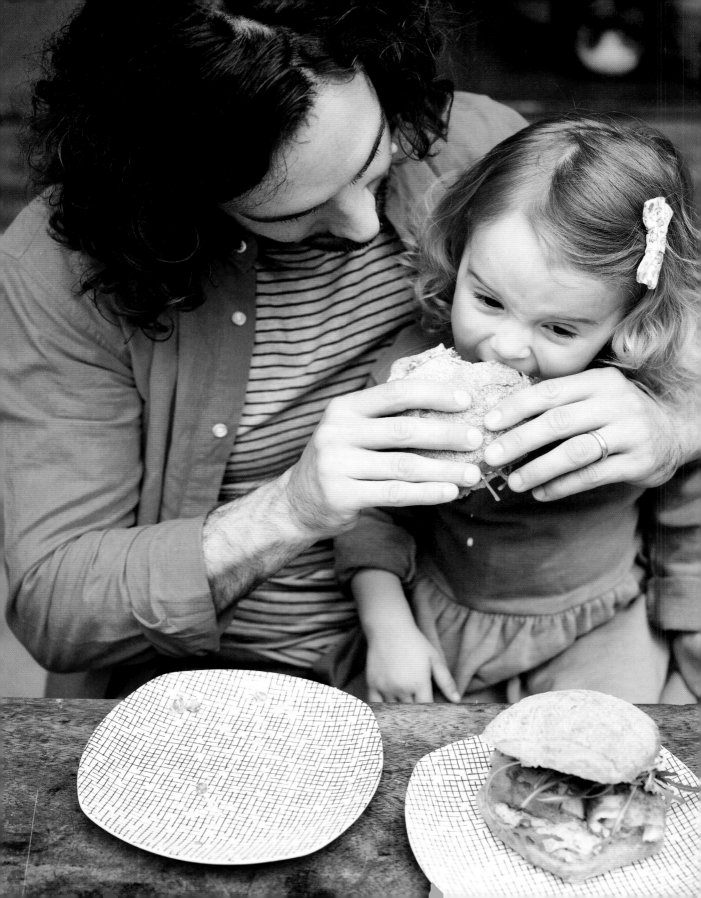

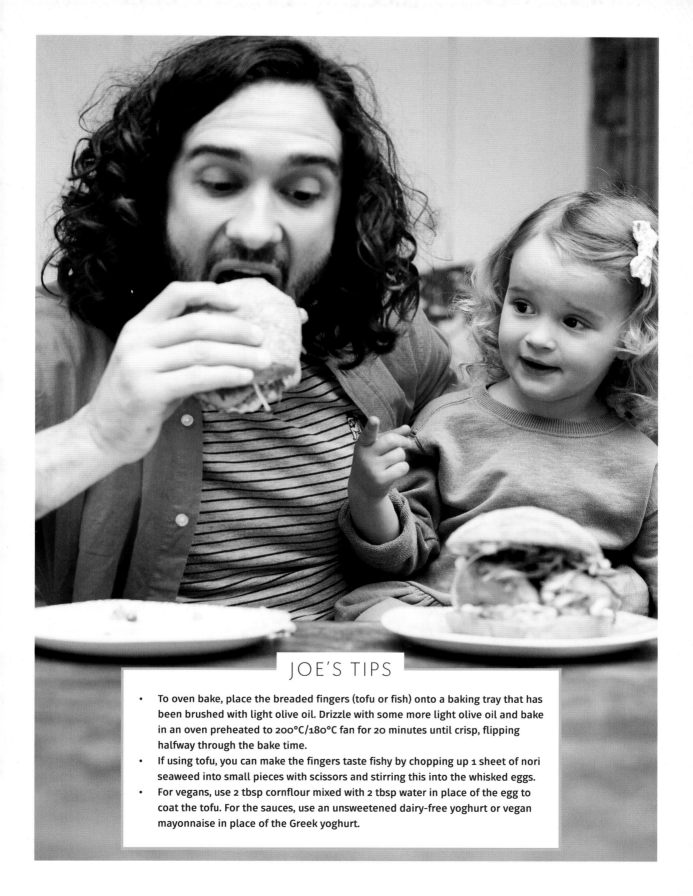

JOE'S TIPS

- To oven bake, place the breaded fingers (tofu or fish) onto a baking tray that has been brushed with light olive oil. Drizzle with some more light olive oil and bake in an oven preheated to 200°C/180°C fan for 20 minutes until crisp, flipping halfway through the bake time.
- If using tofu, you can make the fingers taste fishy by chopping up 1 sheet of nori seaweed into small pieces with scissors and stirring this into the whisked eggs.
- For vegans, use 2 tbsp cornflour mixed with 2 tbsp water in place of the egg to coat the tofu. For the sauces, use an unsweetened dairy-free yoghurt or vegan mayonnaise in place of the Greek yoghurt.

BAKED SPRING ROLLS WITH SESAME & SOY DIPPING SAUCE

Spring rolls are a delicious way to pack a lot of veg into a tasty snack or light meal. My kids love dipping these in the sauce. Using filo pastry and baking them means you get that crispy, crunchy texture without the need for any deep-frying. They make a great party snack, too, for kids and grown-ups.

MAKES 10

1 tsp sesame oil

1 tsp grated fresh ginger

2 garlic cloves, crushed

¼ small head (about 150g) cabbage, thinly sliced

2 medium (about 150g) carrots, coarsely grated

4 spring onions, thinly sliced

100g beansprouts

2 tbsp oyster sauce (or a vegetarian alternative, such as mushroom stir-fry sauce, which is available online)

1 tbsp soy sauce

½ tsp white pepper

1 tsp cornflour

5 sheets of filo pastry

2 tbsp light olive oil

Sesame and Soy Dipping Sauce

1 tsp apple cider vinegar

1 tbsp soy sauce

1 tbsp sesame oil

1 tsp sriracha, or other hot sauce

1 tsp runny honey

1 Heat the sesame oil in a large frying pan over a high heat, add the ginger and garlic and cook for 1–2 minutes to soften. Add the cabbage, carrots, spring onions and beansprouts and continue to cook over a high heat until the veg have completely softened, about 5 minutes. Stir in the oyster sauce, soy sauce and white pepper, then remove from the heat and allow to cool.

2 When cool, sprinkle the cornflour over the mixture and toss everything together with your hands.

3 Preheat the oven to 200°C/180°C fan and line a baking sheet with baking paper.

4 Unwrap the sheets of filo and cut in half widthways so you have 10 rectangles, each measuring about 14 x 26cm. Take one piece of filo, leaving the rest covered with a damp cloth, and place on the work surface so the short edge is facing you. Take around 2 tablespoons of the veg mixture and place it in a line at the bottom of the rectangle, leaving a 3cm border. Fold in the left and right edges of the filo, then, starting at the edge nearest to you, roll up to make a cigar shape. Place onto the baking tray, seam-side down. Repeat until you have used everything up. Brush the rolls with the oil and bake for 15–20 minutes until golden and crisp.

5 Mix all of the dipping sauce ingredients in a small bowl until combined. Serve with the baked spring rolls.

FEEL GOOD FACT

Some studies suggest that regularly eating sesame seeds lowers cholesterol and triglycerides, which are risk factors for heart disease. They are a good source of fibre, plant protein and B vitamins, too.

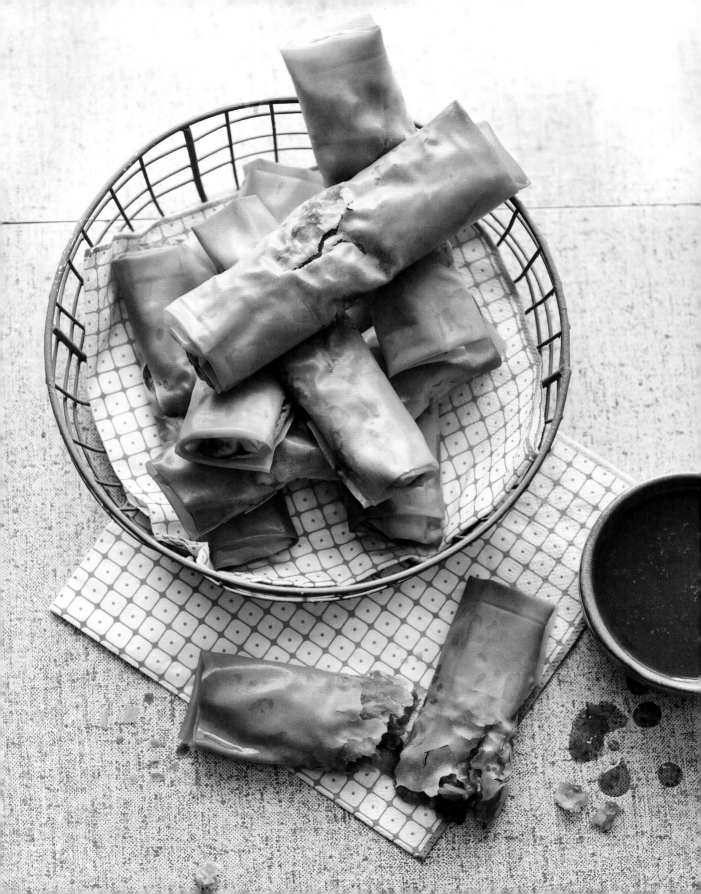

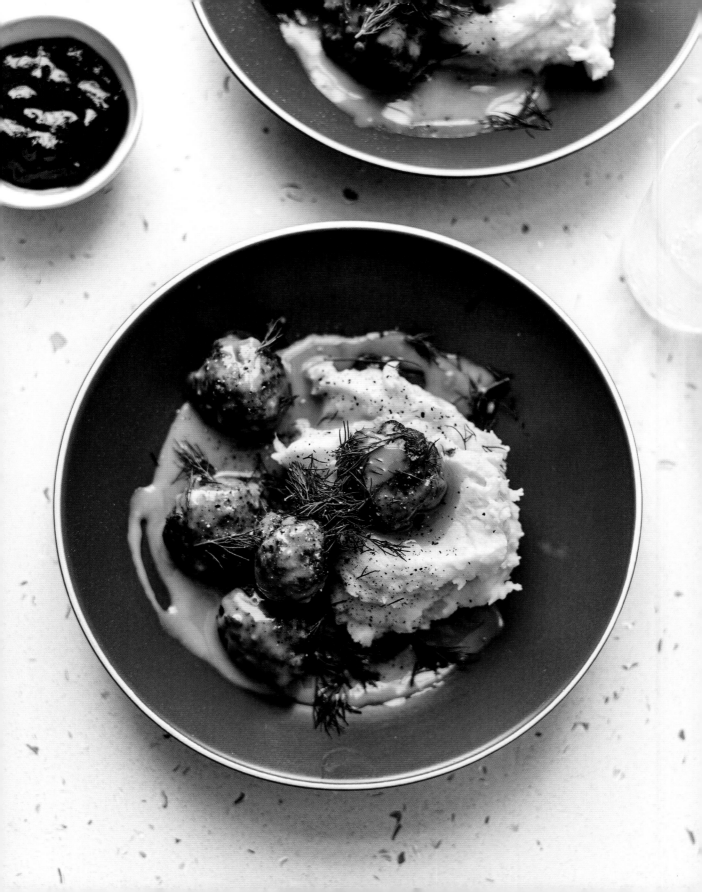

SWEDISH MEATBALLS WITH CELERIAC & POTATO MASH

As a kid, the only reason I was excited to go to IKEA with my mum was because at the end I would always get the Swedish meatballs in the restaurant. So tasty, they bring back good memories. I've given this classic Swedish dish a bit of a twist by adding cannellini beans and chestnut mushrooms, which make the meatballs even juicier and tastier. Wait until you taste the gravy, too! It's a winner!

SERVES 4

Meatballs

300g chestnut mushrooms, chopped

400g tin of cannellini beans, drained

1 onion, diced

400g minced pork

4 tbsp dried breadcrumbs

1 egg, beaten

½ tsp each salt and black pepper

½ tsp ground allspice (optional)

2–3 tbsp light olive oil, for cooking

Celeriac Potato Mash

600g potatoes (about 3 medium), peeled and cut into quarters

350g celeriac (about ½ head), peeled and cut into 3cm chunks

30g butter

2 tbsp reduced-fat crème fraîche

salt and freshly ground black pepper

Creamy Gravy

2 tbsp unsalted butter

2½ tbsp plain white flour

500ml beef stock

¼ tsp ground white pepper

2 tbsp reduced-fat crème fraîche

2–4 tsp soy sauce

To Serve (optional)

chopped dill

cranberry sauce or lingonberry jam

1 Place the mushrooms in a dry frying pan and cook over a medium heat, stirring occasionally, until they've released all their liquid and are starting to brown. Tip them into the bowl of a food processor along with the cannellini beans and onion, and pulse until you get a slightly chunky paste.

2 Scrape the mixture into a medium bowl and add the remaining meatball ingredients, except the oil, and squish everything together with your hands until well combined.

3 Heat 1 tablespoon of the oil in a large frying pan over a medium-low heat. Shape the pork mixture into small, bite-sized balls and place them in the pan, leaving a bit of room between each meatball. You will most likely have to cook them in a few batches to avoid crowding the pan. Cook, turning frequently, until golden brown all over and cooked through.

4 Meanwhile, make the mash. Put the potato and celeriac chunks in a large saucepan and cover with cold water. Bring to the boil, then cook for a further 15–20 minutes until both are soft. Drain and return to the pan, then mash with a potato masher until mostly smooth. Add the butter and crème fraîche and mash through. Season with salt and pepper, to taste.

5 For the gravy, melt the butter in a medium pan over a high heat. Add the flour and stir for 1 minute. Reduce the heat to medium-low and gradually whisk in the beef stock until smooth. Mix in the white pepper and cook until the sauce thickens. Stir in the crème fraîche, then add soy sauce, to taste.

6 Serve the meatballs warm with the mash and gravy, sprinkled with dill and maybe a bit of cranberry sauce or lingonberry jam on the side, too. You can make any of the components here ahead of time and store them in the fridge for up to 3 days. Just warm them up before serving.

THAI GREEN CHICKEN & PEA CURRY

Thai green curry is one of my favourite things to make, because it's so tasty and reminds me of my time travelling around Thailand. Pre-made curry pastes make life easier and keep this recipe nice and simple. Serve with brown rice for some wholegrain goodness (although white rice is fine, too).

SERVES 4

1 tbsp coconut oil

2 chicken breasts, cut into 3cm chunks

2 onions, diced

4 garlic cloves, crushed

2 tbsp grated fresh ginger

4 tbsp green Thai curry paste

400g tin of coconut milk

300ml chicken or vegetable stock

300g frozen peas

175g baby corn, cut into 2cm chunks

200g Tenderstem broccoli, stems roughly chopped

soy sauce, to taste (optional)

To Serve

500g cooked brown basmati rice

1 lime, cut into wedges

1 Heat half of the coconut oil in a deep frying pan over a medium heat, add the chicken pieces and cook until browned and no longer pink in the middle. Remove to a plate.

2 Add the remaining oil to the pan, followed by the onions, and cook for 5–7 minutes until softened, then stir in the garlic and ginger for 1 minute. Add the curry paste and cook for a further 2 minutes. Pour in the coconut milk, stock and peas, then heat until it starts to gently simmer.

3 Remove from the heat and blitz until smooth, either using a hand blender directly in the pan or using a free-standing blender.

4 Pour the mixture back into the pan, if needed, and return to the heat. Add the corn, broccoli and cooked chicken and bring back to a simmer. Cook for 4–6 minutes until the vegetables are cooked to your liking. Taste and season with soy sauce, if needed.

5 Serve with the cooked rice, with lime wedges on the side for squeezing over.

FEEL GOOD FACT

Heart-healthy peas provide the sweetness in this classic Thai curry sauce instead of the more usual sugar.

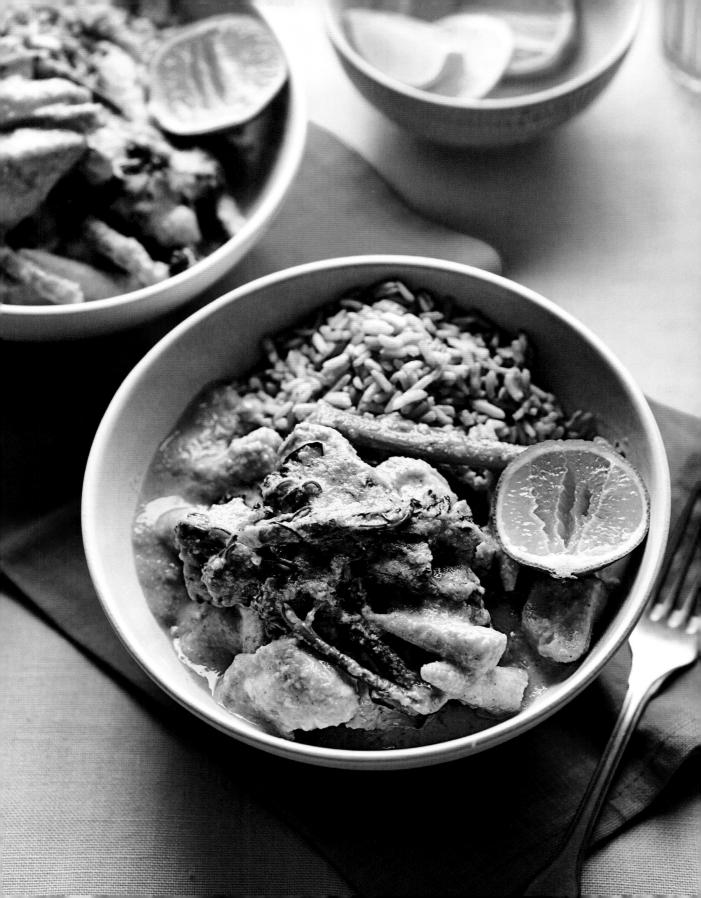

ONE-POT LAMB & VEGETABLE BIRYANI

This is a proper feel good, home-style, pot-on-the-table family dinner. Although this classic Indian dish is started off on the hob, it is finished in the oven, giving you a bit of a break from the cooking while the oven does the rest of the work. I use brown basmati rice, but white basmati is fine, too. A very, very tasty recipe!

SERVES 4

100g natural yoghurt

1 tbsp grated fresh ginger

2 garlic cloves, crushed

2 tsp garam masala

½ tsp ground cinnamon

½ tsp chilli powder

½ tsp ground turmeric

½ tsp freshly ground black pepper

½ tsp salt, plus extra to taste

2 handfuls of fresh coriander, finely chopped

handful of mint leaves, finely chopped

400g diced lamb shoulder (or quick-cook or loin)

1½ tbsp coconut oil

3 small or 2 medium onions, thinly sliced

½ head of cauliflower, cut into small florets

100g green beans, trimmed

150g frozen peas

500g cooked brown basmati rice

handful of cashew nuts, roughly chopped

handful of raisins

1 Preheat the oven to 200°C/180°C fan.

2 Combine the yoghurt, ginger, garlic, spices and salt in a large bowl. Add half of the coriander (reserving the rest for garnish), the mint and diced lamb, and stir to coat. Set aside to marinate for 30 minutes.

3 Heat the coconut oil in an ovenproof casserole dish over a medium-low heat, add the onions with a pinch of salt and sauté for 15 minutes, until golden, then remove them to a plate.

4 Add the cauliflower and green beans to the dish and sauté over a medium heat until browned, then stir in the peas for a minute so that they defrost. Remove all the vegetables to a separate plate.

5 Add the marinated lamb to the dish and cook for a few minutes until the meat is no longer pink. Add the vegetables (not the onions) back in, stir, then remove from the heat.

6 Scoop out half of the mixture to a plate and layer half of the cooked rice over what remains in the casserole dish. Return the mixture you just scooped out back into the dish and layer over the rice. Cover this layer with the remaining rice. Cover with a lid (or tightly with foil) and bake for 20 minutes.

7 Uncover the dish and check the seasoning. Garnish the biryani with the cooked onions, reserved coriander, cashews and raisins, and serve.

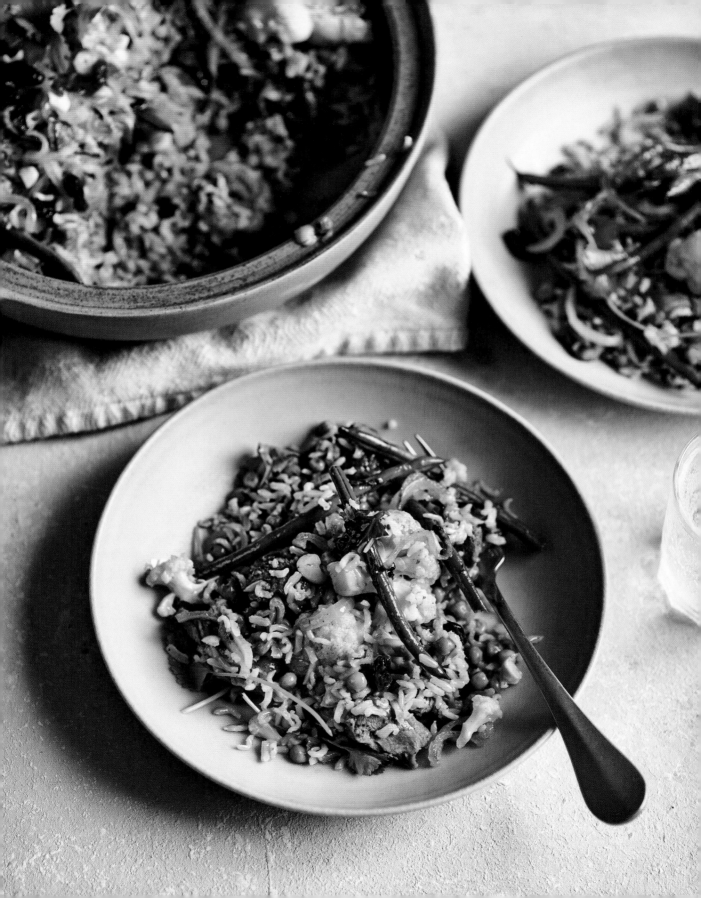

NO-KNEAD FRYING-PAN PIZZA

Making your own pizza is SO rewarding and so much fun, especially with kids! The nutritious wholemeal flour dough is so easy to throw together and the no-cook tomato sauce is also incredibly quick to make, so you have more time to have fun adding your favourite toppings. No need for a professional pizza oven – an oven-safe frying pan and your grill are just fine.

MAKES 4

Pizza Dough

350ml water

½ tsp fast-action dried yeast

250g wholemeal bread flour

250g white bread flour, plus extra
    for dusting

1 tsp table salt

olive oil, for greasing

Tomato Sauce

1 tbsp extra-virgin olive oil

400g tin of peeled plum tomatoes

1 garlic clove, crushed

1 tbsp balsamic vinegar

1 tsp dried oregano

pinch of salt

Toppings

2 x 125g balls of fresh mozzarella, drained
    and cut into small chunks

30g Parmesan cheese, finely grated

handful of fresh basil, torn

Optional Extra Toppings

sun-dried tomatoes, pitted olives,
    sweetcorn, chargrilled peppers, steamed
    broccoli florets, roasted butternut squash
    chunks, shredded cooked chicken breast,
    salami, rocket, artichoke hearts, pesto

1 Make the pizza dough on the morning of the day you want to eat it. Add the water to a medium bowl and sprinkle over the yeast. Let it sit for 5 minutes, then stir in all the flour and the salt. Mix with a spoon to get a shaggy dough, then use your hands to mix until you have a soft, sticky dough. Divide the dough into quarters and roll each piece into a ball.

2 Pour some olive oil into a deep baking dish and spread it around to coat the base and sides. Put the balls of dough in the dish, spacing them at least 7cm apart (you may need another dish if they won't all fit). Drizzle a bit more oil on top and rub it over the entire surface of each dough ball. Cover the dish with a small, clean bag (which can be re-used) or a piece of clingfilm, and set aside somewhere cool, out of direct sunlight, for 8 hours (see also my Tip, overleaf).

3 For the tomato sauce, combine all the ingredients in a bowl. Use your hands to squish everything together and to break up the tomatoes into very small chunks. Refrigerate until needed.

4 When you're ready to eat, sprinkle your work surface with flour. Gently remove a dough ball from the dish, leaving the rest covered, and place onto the flour. Sprinkle some more flour on top. Use your hands to gently pat down the centre of the ball, leaving a rim a few centimetres thick. Gently stretch and pull the dough to form a circle about 25cm in diameter, trying to leave the rim slightly thicker than the middle. If this is too fiddly, use a rolling pin to roll the dough into a circle, dusting the top and underside with flour, as needed, to prevent sticking.

5 Place a rack into the top part of your oven and preheat the oven on the grill setting.

Continues overleaf

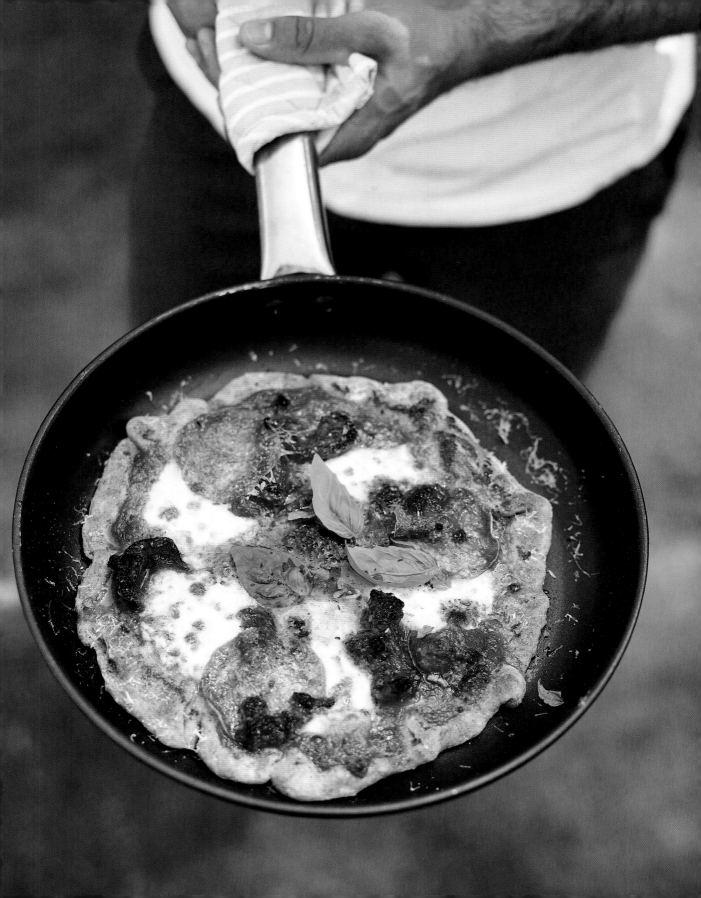

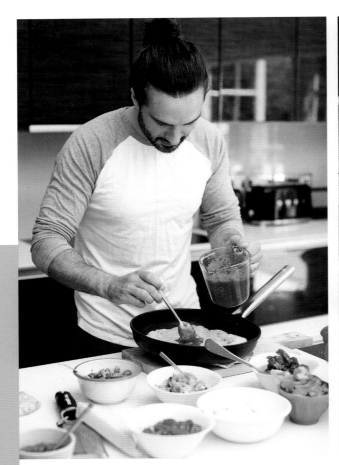

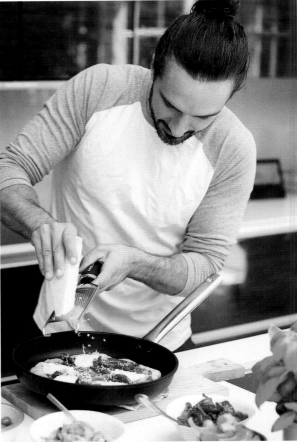

JOE'S TIP

This easy no-knead pizza dough needs hardly any hands-on time. Just mix it and let it sit during the day, perhaps while you're at work, then it's ready to use in the evening. If you need to leave the dough a little longer, pop it into the fridge after the 8 hours is up – it can stay there for up to a day.

6 Heat a large frying pan over a high heat on the stove. Once the pan is hot, add the stretched circle of dough and cook until it starts to bubble on top and the underside is golden. Turn the heat down to low and spread a few tablespoons of the tomato sauce onto the pizza – you don't want a super-thick layer of sauce or it'll be too wet.

7 Remove the pan from the heat and sprinkle some of the mozzarella on top. Add any other toppings you like, then finish with a little sprinkle of Parmesan.

8 Place the pan into the oven under the grill, with the oven door open and the handle sticking out. Cook until the cheese has melted and the crust is starting to brown, around 4 minutes.

9 Remove from the oven (use oven mitts or a tea towel as the handle will be hot) and slide the pizza out onto a board. Garnish with the torn basil and serve.

10 Repeat until all the pizzas are cooked.

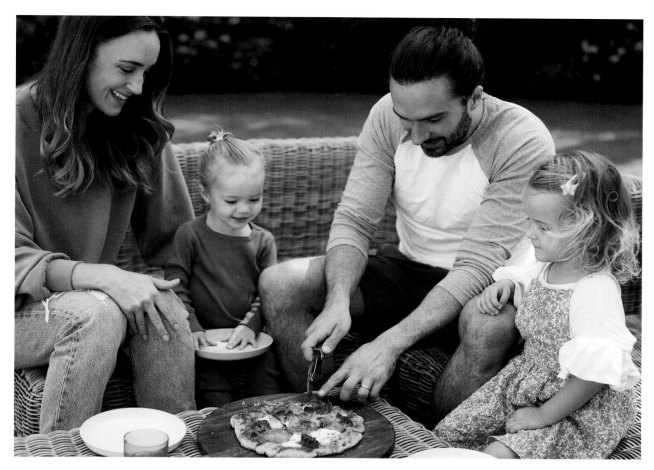
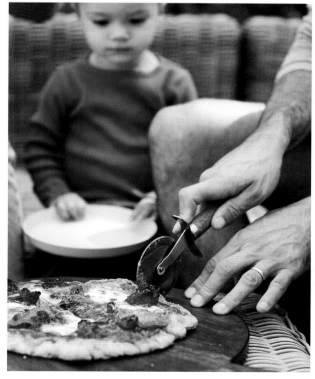
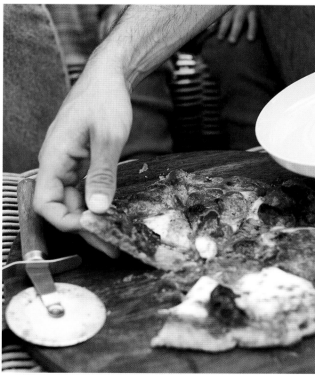

SPICY 'SHROOM & LENTIL TACOS WITH FRESH SALSA

This veggie taco recipe is a taste sensation, especially with the charred pineapple salsa. The sauce is full of flavour from the spices and mushrooms, so you won't miss the meat. I've added lentils to fill them out and bring some extra protein.

SERVES 4

600g chestnut mushrooms, chopped

pinch of salt

2 tbsp light olive oil

2 red onions, diced

100g (6 tbsp) tomato purée concentrate (tomato paste)

2 x 400g tins of lentils, drained and rinsed

1 tbsp ground cumin

2 tsp smoked paprika

2 tsp garlic granules or 2 garlic cloves, crushed

½–1 tsp chilli flakes

2–3 tbsp soy sauce, to taste

2 tbsp sriracha, or other hot sauce (optional)

Charred Pineapple and Tomato Salsa

300g frozen pineapple chunks

200g tomatoes (I use regular tomatoes, but you could use cherry tomatoes if you like)

juice of ½ lemon or lime

handful of fresh coriander, chopped

1 shallot or ½ red onion, finely diced

pinch of salt

To Serve

8–10 small tortillas

100g feta cheese, crumbled (omit if vegan)

handful of fresh coriander, chopped

lime wedges

1 Add the mushrooms to a large, dry frying pan with the salt, and cook over a medium heat until they've released their liquid and are starting to brown. Add the oil and onions and cook for about 10 minutes, stirring occasionally, until the onions are softened and starting to caramelise.

2 Add the tomato purée and cook until it darkens, then mix in the drained lentils, cumin, paprika, garlic, chilli flakes, soy sauce and sriracha (if using). Stir until warmed through, then remove from the heat. Taste and add more soy sauce, if needed.

3 For the salsa, place the pineapple chunks in a dry frying pan or griddle pan. Cook over a high heat until the pineapple starts to char underneath, then flip the chunks and repeat on the other sides. Once charred all over, remove them from the pan to a chopping board and roughly chop into small pieces, then scrape into a bowl. Cut the tomatoes into small chunks and add to the bowl of pineapple. Stir in the lemon or lime juice, chopped coriander, shallot or onion and the salt.

4 Warm the tortillas according to the packet instructions.

5 Top each warmed tortilla with some of the spicy mushroom and lentil mixture and finish with pineapple salsa, crumbled feta (if using) and chopped coriander. Serve with lime wedges.

VARIATIONS

- If you don't like lentils, feel free to replace them with your favourite tinned bean. Black beans or kidney beans are particularly good here.
- You can use fresh pineapple instead of the frozen chunks.
- If you don't like pineapple, just leave it out and increase the quantity of tomatoes to 500g.

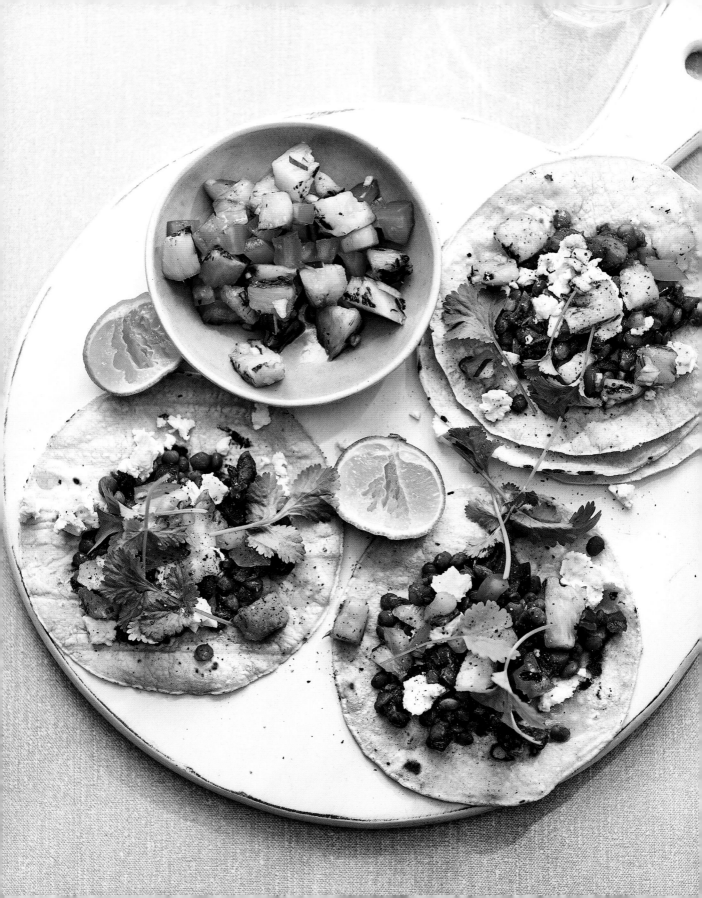

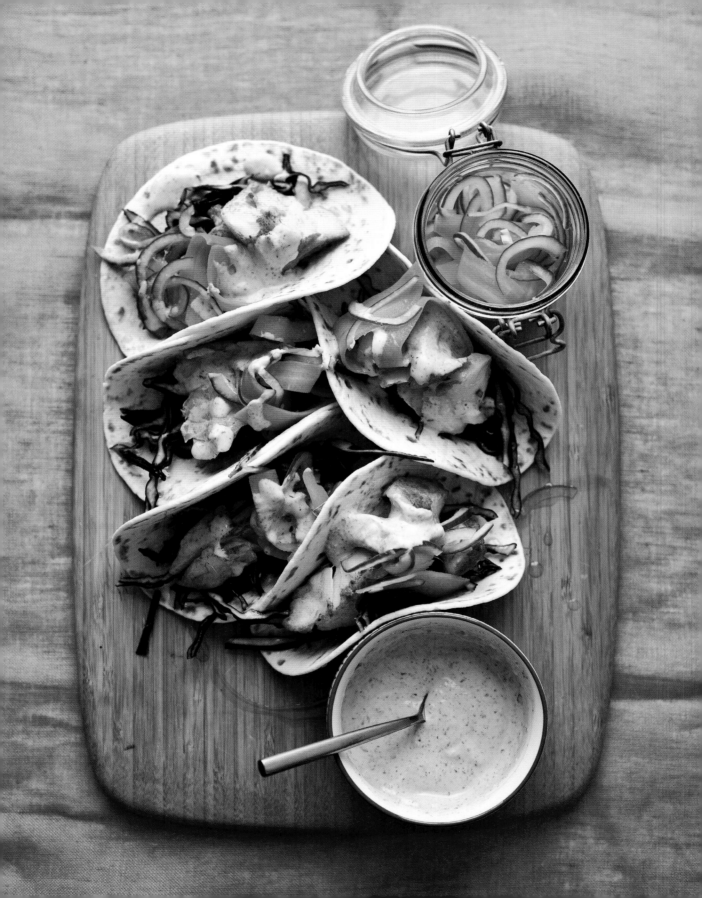

SPICED FISH TACOS

Tacos are a really fun way of eating together, and perfect for weeknight suppers. I like to cook and prepare all of the ingredients and put them on the table in little bowls, then let the kids go to town on their very own creations. This cod is only lightly spiced, so it's great for the kids to try, too. Messy but very fun!

SERVES 4

Quick Pickles

1 red onion, thinly sliced

1 carrot, peeled into ribbons

60ml apple cider vinegar

40ml water

1 tbsp sugar

1 tsp salt

Spiced Cod

1 tsp smoked paprika

½ tsp ground cumin

¼ tsp cayenne pepper

1 tsp salt, or to taste

½ tsp black pepper

4 x 140g skinless cod fillets

1 tbsp light olive oil

Dressing

150g 0%-fat Greek yoghurt

1 garlic clove, crushed

pinch of salt

3 tbsp extra-virgin olive oil

30g fresh coriander, roughly chopped

1 tbsp lime juice

¼–½ jalapeño, seeds removed, chopped

½ tsp honey

To Serve

12 small tortillas (preferably wholemeal)

¼ red cabbage, very thinly sliced

1 Start with the quick pickles. Place the thinly sliced onion and carrot ribbons in a medium bowl.

2 Heat the apple cider vinegar, water, sugar and salt in a small pan over a high heat until steaming. Pour the hot mixture over the onion and carrot in the bowl and set aside for at least 15 minutes until the onion is bright pink.

3 Meanwhile, make the spiced cod. Mix the smoked paprika, cumin and cayenne with the salt and pepper in a small bowl. Lay the cod fillets out on a chopping board and sprinkle with the spice mix, turning over to coat the other sides as well.

4 Heat the oil in a non-stick frying pan over a medium heat. Add the spiced cod and cook on both sides until it flakes apart easily. Remove from the heat and flake the fish. Taste and season with more salt, if needed.

5 Blitz together all the dressing ingredients in a food processor or using a hand blender until smooth. If you don't have a blender, finely chop the coriander and jalapeño and mix everything together in a medium bowl. Thin the dressing with a couple of tablespoons or so of water until thick but drizzleable.

6 Warm the tortillas according to the packet instructions.

7 Serve the cod in the warmed tortillas with the sliced cabbage, pickles and a drizzle of dressing.

ROASTED BRUSSELS SPROUT CARBONARA

This is such a bangin' recipe. Roasted Brussels sprouts are a game-changer. They take on a totally new flavour and texture to the smelly ones your granny used to boil in water. They become sweet and nutty and crispy, and are honestly amazing. I never thought I'd ever say that about sprouts, but it's true. I think you'll love this one!

SERVES 4

500g Brussels sprouts, halved
1 tbsp light olive oil
160g pancetta cubes
300g wholemeal spaghetti
4 egg yolks
50g Parmesan cheese, finely grated
salt and freshly ground black pepper

1 Preheat the oven to 220°C/200°C fan.

2 Toss the sprouts with the oil on a large baking tray. Sprinkle the pancetta cubes over the sprouts. Roast for 20–25 minutes until the pancetta is crisp and the sprouts are golden.

3 Meanwhile, bring a large pan of salted water to the boil, add the spaghetti and cook according to the packet instructions.

4 As the spaghetti is boiling, place the egg yolks into a large bowl along with the Parmesan and a few grindings of black pepper. Stir together.

5 Use tongs to transfer the cooked spaghetti straight from the pan to the bowl with the eggy cheese mixture and quickly toss together, loosening with a splash of pasta water from the pan as needed. The hot pasta will cook the egg yolks and melt the cheese to make a creamy sauce.

6 Divide the pasta between plates and top with the roasted sprouts and pancetta.

FEEL GOOD FACT

Carbonara seems like it contains loads of cheese and cream, but in reality it doesn't have much at all. By using Parmesan, which has a strong flavour, you still get that cheesy hit from just a small amount. The creaminess comes from the egg yolks. Sprouts are high in fibre and rich in vitamins C and K.

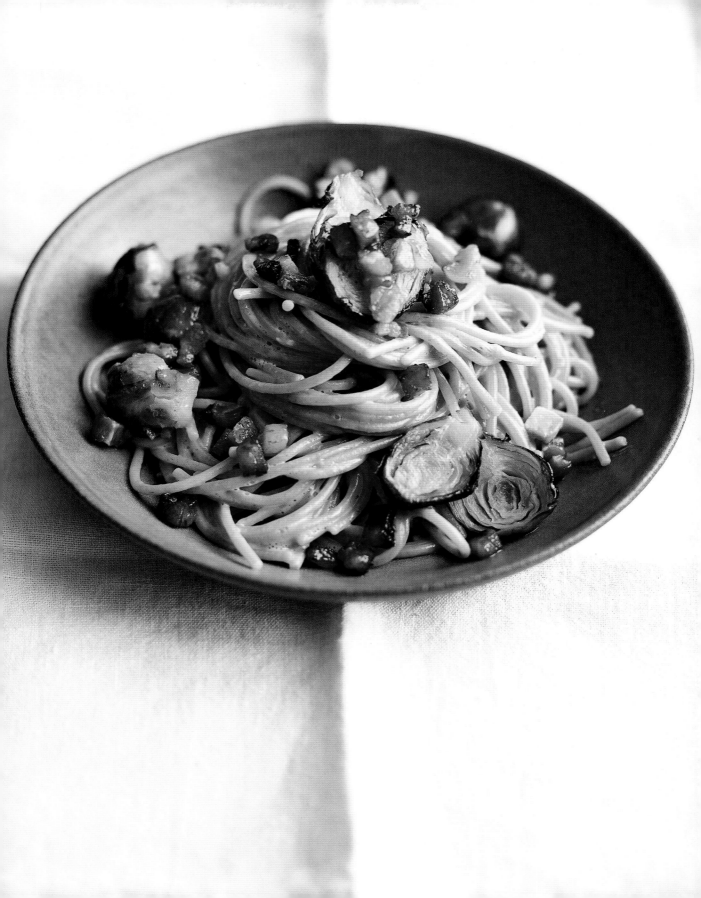

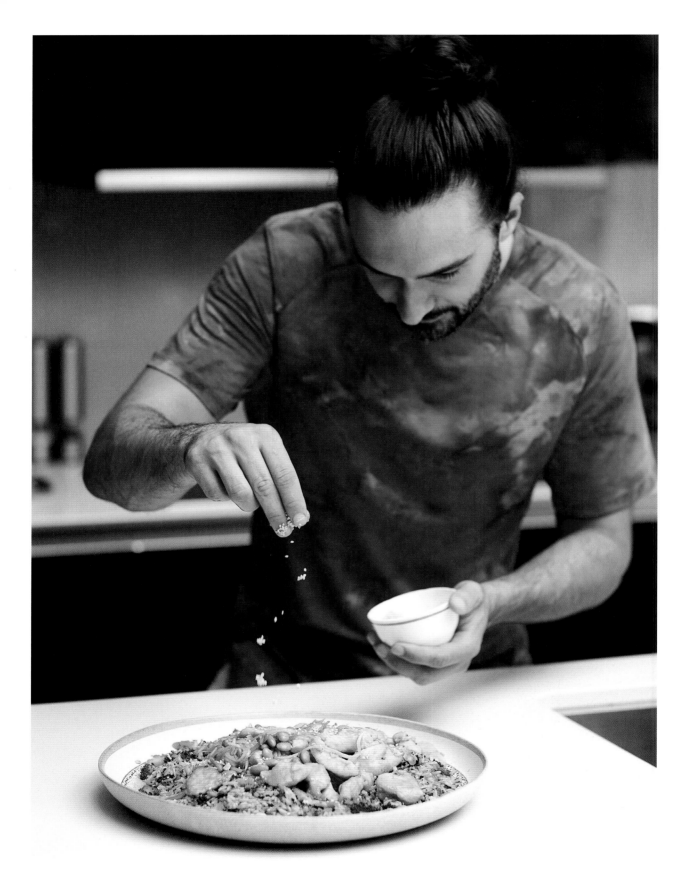

5

SPEEDY

quick weeknight suppers
to fill you up fast

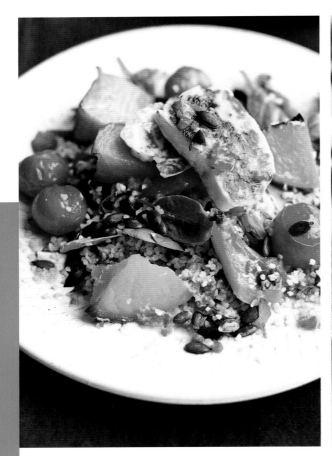
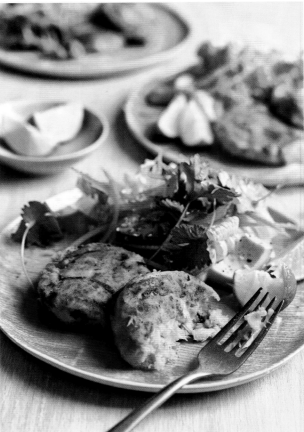

Weeknights are always so busy, it's great to have some super-quick recipes up your sleeve. Ones that you know you can whip up in a flash and that everyone in the family will love. Or sometimes, you just want something where the prep is simple and quick and then you can just leave it to cook and forget about it for a while, while you get on with the business of a hectic family evening. I've got you covered either way.

I've got loads of my favourite speedy ingredients in this chapter: gnocchi, pasta, eggs… And some great new ways of giving store-bought family favourites a new twist, such as sausages or filled pasta.

I'm a huge fan of a traybake – just chuck it all in and bang it in the oven for a bit. So, I've made sure to include plenty of them here. The sausage traybake on

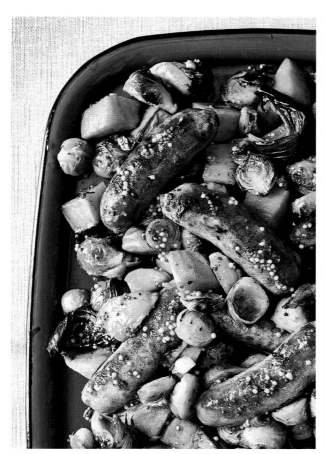

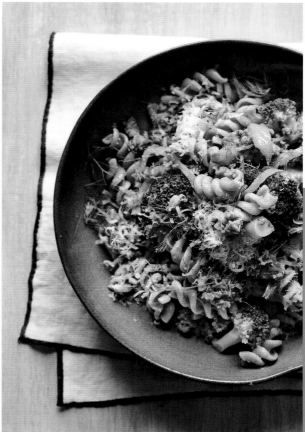

page 171 is wicked – I do hope you give it a go. And who doesn't love a pasta bake? Try the one on page 186 – it'll have you looking at store-bought filled pasta in a whole new way.

Stir-fries are also big news in my house. There's nothing healthier, tastier and quicker to whip up. I've got loads for you to try here.

Or how about some freezer-friendly fishcakes (page 168)? Make a big batch in advance and then you'll have them ready to whip out whenever the going gets tough. My kids love them, so I always make sure I have some ready-made for a quick meal.

SPEEDY

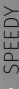

BAKED FETA WITH ROASTED VEG & PESTO DRESSING

Baking a whole block of feta like this is so easy – it becomes soft and creamy and you then simply stir it into roasted veg for a delicious lunch or dinner. With skin-on new potatoes and plenty of colourful veg, this has everything you need for a well-balanced meal.

SERVES 4

800g new potatoes, halved

2 red peppers, seeds removed, cut into strips

350g cherry tomatoes, halved

4 sprigs of thyme

2 tbsp light olive oil

pinch of salt

200g Brussels sprouts, halved

200g feta cheese

Pesto Dressing

4 tbsp basil pesto

1 tbsp lemon juice

1 tbsp extra-virgin olive oil

1 Preheat the oven to 200°C/180°C fan.

2 Place the potatoes in a medium saucepan and just cover with water. Pop a lid on and place over a high heat. Once the water is boiling, remove the lid and simmer the potatoes for 6–8 minutes until tender.

3 Drain the potatoes and tumble onto a large, rimmed baking tray along with the peppers, tomatoes, thyme sprigs, light olive oil and salt. Roast for 30 minutes, tossing halfway through, until softened and starting to brown.

4 Remove the tray from the oven, add the Brussels sprouts and mix them in, then nestle the block of feta cheese into the middle. Bake for a further 20 minutes until the vegetables are golden around the edges and the feta is soft.

5 Mix together the dressing ingredients in a jar or small bowl, pour over the contents of the tray and serve.

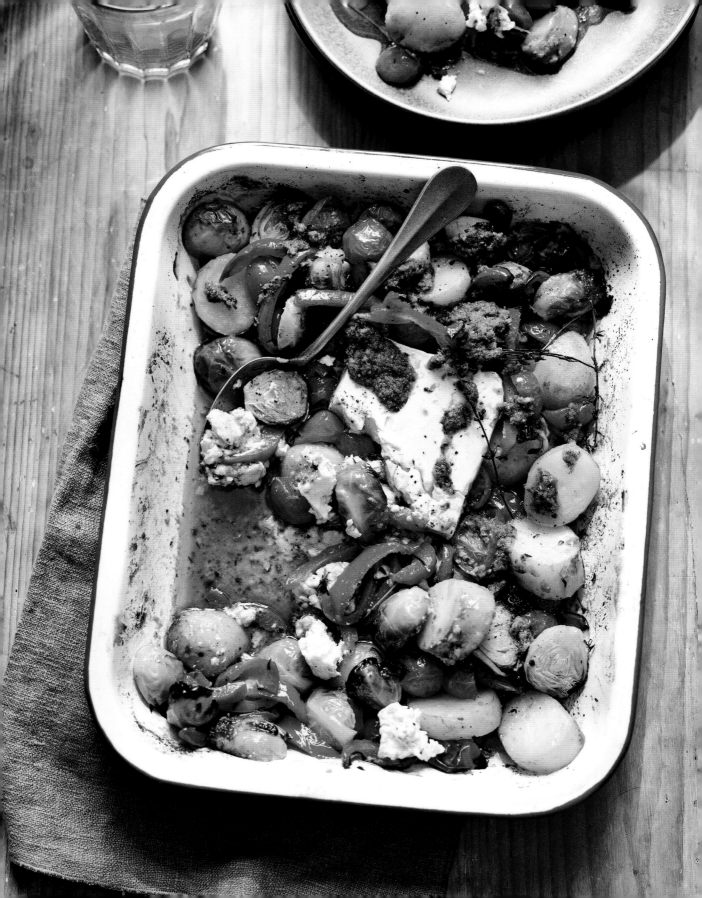

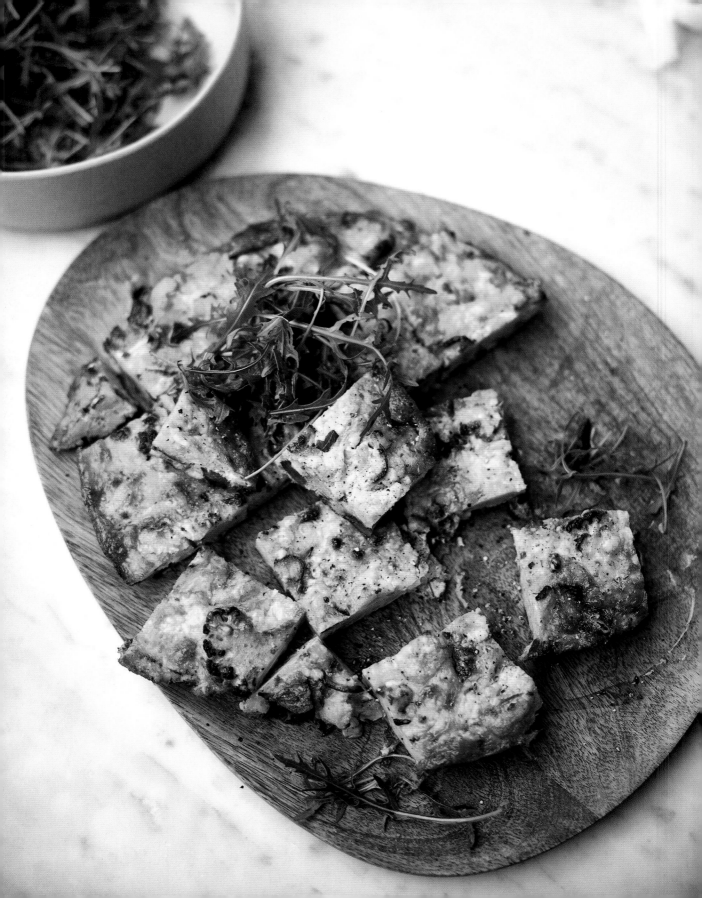

CAULIFLOWER, CHORIZO & CORN FRITTATA

I think frittatas are wicked because they are so quick and simple to make and you can literally throw anything you like in them. They also keep really well in the fridge for the next day, so they are great to batch cook. This one gets a kick of flavour from the chorizo, but if you want to keep it veggie you can just leave the chorizo out.

SERVES 4

75g chorizo sausage, roughly chopped

1 red onion, thinly sliced

1 small cauliflower, cut into small florets

175g frozen sweetcorn

8 eggs

pinch each of salt and freshly ground black pepper

80g Cheddar cheese, grated

handful of rocket leaves, to serve

1 Place a large, non-stick oven-safe frying pan over a medium-high heat and add the chorizo chunks. Cook until the fat has rendered from the chorizo and it's crispy. Remove the chorizo from the pan to a plate, leaving as much fat as possible in the pan.

2 Add the onion to the pan, reduce the heat to medium-low and sauté until softened, around 5 minutes. Next, add the cauliflower florets and sauté for another 5 minutes until browned. Stir in the frozen corn until it defrosts, then mix the chorizo back in.

3 Meanwhile, preheat the grill to high.

4 Whisk the eggs with the salt and pepper in a bowl. Pour the egg over the contents of the pan and sprinkle with the grated cheese. Cook until golden underneath, then pop under the grill (with the pan handle sticking out) until the cheese is melted and the egg is set.

5 Loosen the frittata from the pan with a spatula, then slide it out onto a serving platter and garnish with the rocket.

JOE'S TIP

Serve with some warm crusty bread or a side of soup to make this a more filling meal.

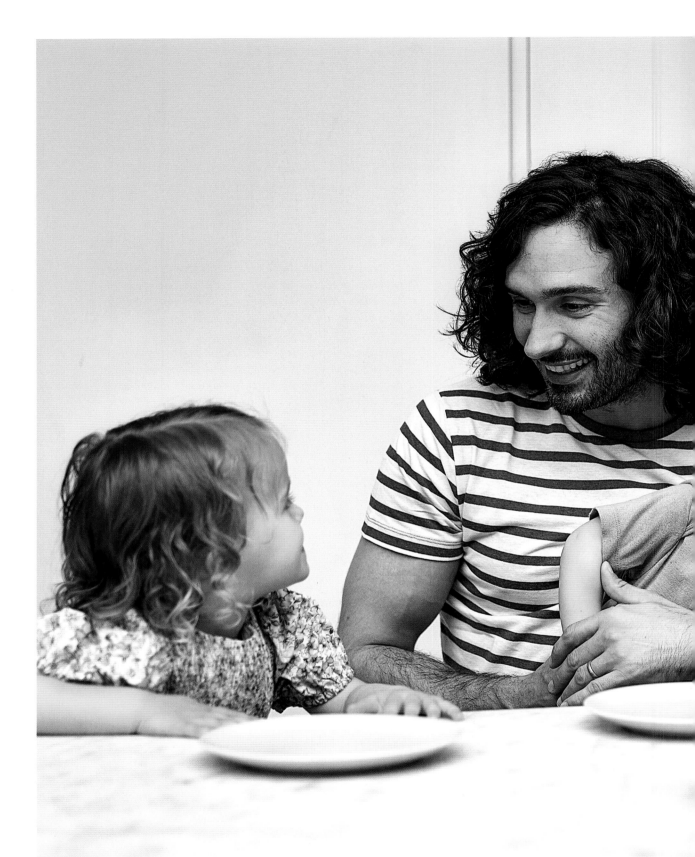

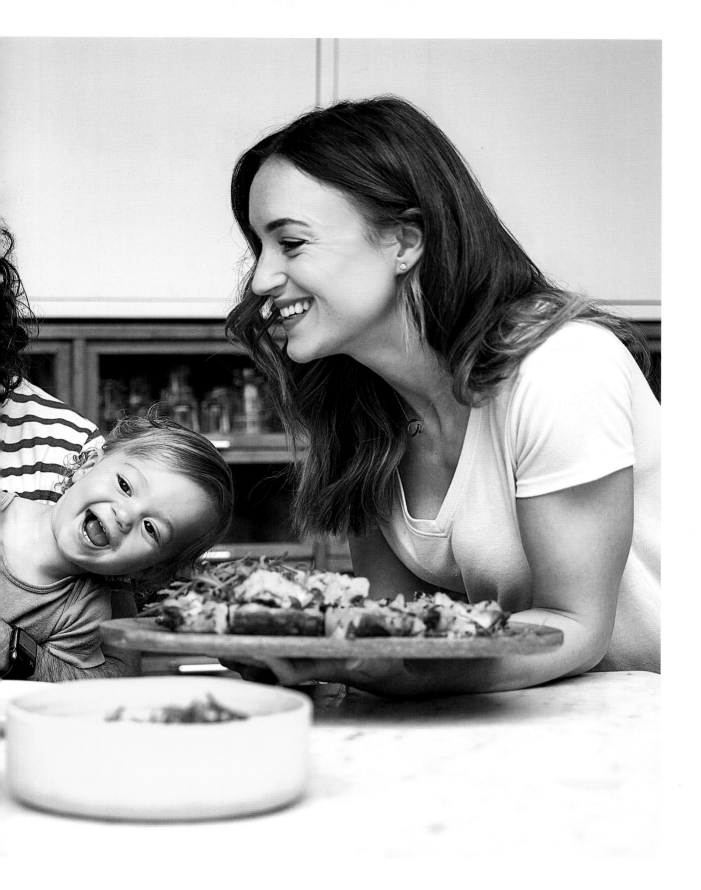

GINGER & CORIANDER SALMON FISHCAKES

Fishcakes are an amazing invention – you can just fold in your favourite herbs and spices to any fish you like. Here, I use salmon with ginger, coriander and spring onion, which is so fresh and delicious. These are also freezer-friendly, so are ideal for batch cooking or for prepping ahead. You can heat them up in the oven for a quick dinner.

SERVES 4

400g skin-on salmon fillets

500g potatoes, peeled and cut into 4cm chunks

30g fresh coriander, roughly chopped

2 garlic cloves, crushed

2 tbsp soy sauce

1 tbsp sriracha, or other hot sauce (optional)

1 tbsp grated fresh ginger

3 spring onions, finely sliced

1 egg white

4 tbsp plain flour

about 2 tbsp coconut oil

To Serve

1 head of romaine lettuce, leaves separated and washed

1 carrot, peeled into ribbons

1 avocado, stone removed, peeled, diced

juice of 1 lime

1½ tsp runny honey

pinch of salt

2 tbsp sesame seeds

1 Preheat the oven to 200°C/180°C fan and line a baking tray with baking paper.

2 Place the salmon on the baking tray and bake for 15 minutes. Allow to cool slightly before removing and discarding the skin.

3 Place the potatoes in a medium saucepan, cover with cold water and bring to the boil over a high heat. Reduce to a simmer and cook for 20 minutes, or until very tender. Drain and return the potatoes to the pan, then mash until smooth.

4 Tip the mashed potato into a large bowl and add the coriander, garlic, soy sauce, sriracha (if using), ginger, spring onions and egg white. Mix together to combine. Flake the fish and fold in.

5 Divide the fish mixture into 12 balls, flatten into patties and dredge in the flour, dusting off any excess.

6 Heat 1 tablespoon of the coconut oil in a medium non-stick frying pan over a medium heat. Add a few patties to the pan and cook until golden underneath, then flip and cook the other side until golden. Remove to a plate. Fry the remaining patties, adding more coconut oil to the pan as needed.

7 Chop the lettuce leaves and add to a bowl with the carrot ribbons and diced avocado. Add the lime juice, honey, salt and sesame seeds, then toss together to coat.

8 Serve the fishcakes warm with the salad on the side.

JOE'S TIP

Freeze the fish cakes after frying and cooling. Reheat from frozen at 200°C/180°C fan for 15–20 minutes until piping hot throughout.

SPEEDY

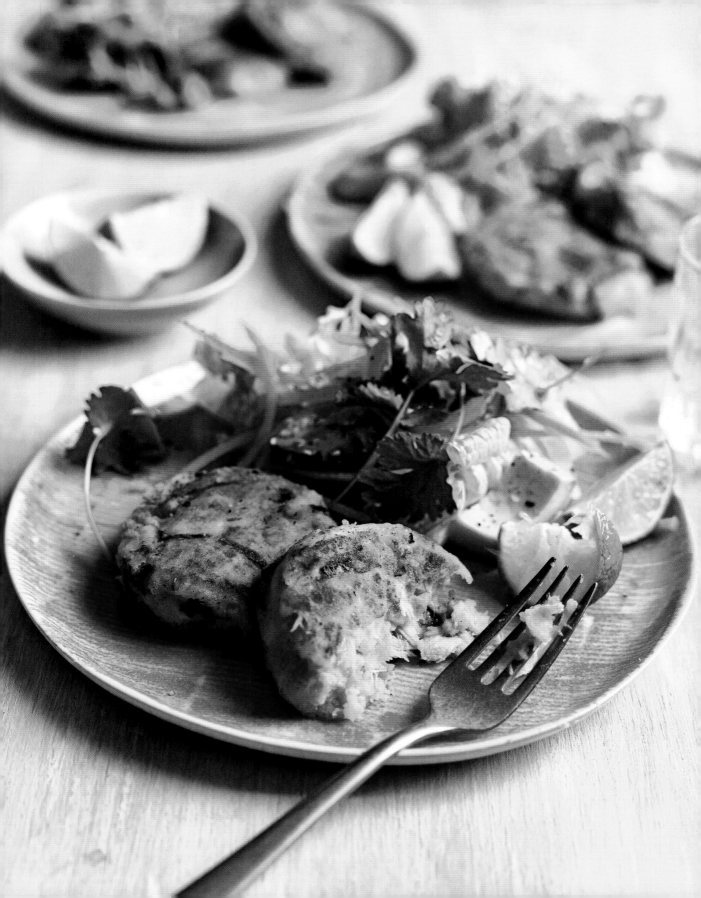

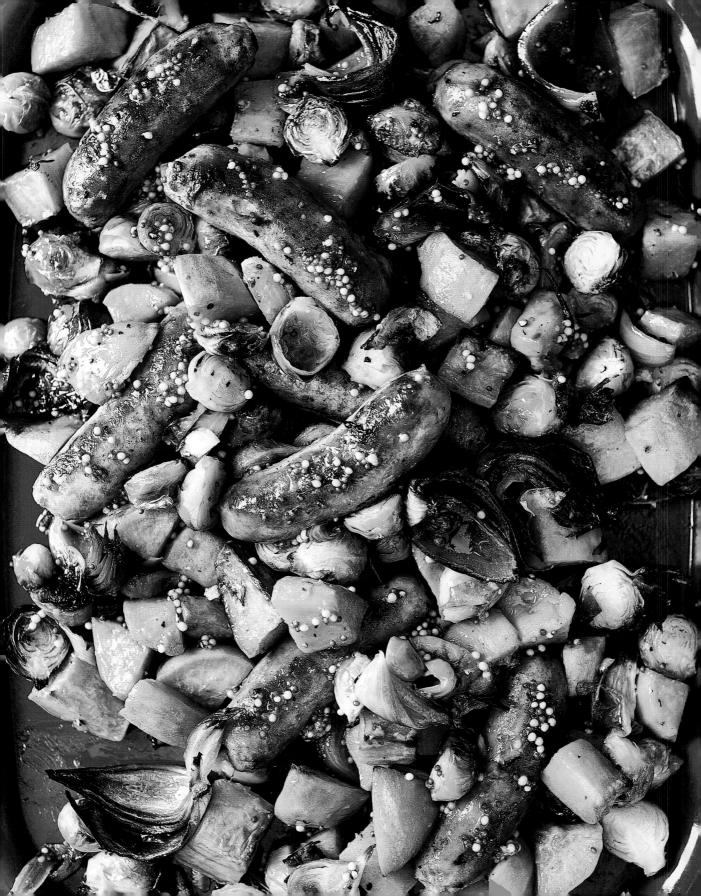

SAUSAGE, SWEET POTATO & MUSTARD TRAYBAKE

Simple but satisfying, this traybake is so easy to chuck in the oven and so tasty! It's ideal any night of the week. It's got roasted sprouts and sweet potatoes, too, so there's loads of goodness as well as lots of flavour from the mustard and sausages.

SERVES 4

4 medium sweet potatoes, peeled and cut into 3cm cubes

2 red onions, peeled and cut into 6 wedges

2 sprigs of rosemary

2 tbsp olive oil

8 pork sausages

500g Brussels sprouts, halved

Dressing

1 tbsp wholegrain mustard

juice of 1 lemon

1 garlic clove, finely grated

pinch of salt

pinch of black pepper

1 Preheat the oven to 220°C/200°C fan.

2 Spread the sweet potatoes, red onions and rosemary over a large, rimmed baking tray. Drizzle with the olive oil and toss together to coat, then lay the sausages on top.

3 Bake for 20 minutes until the sweet potatoes are starting to soften. Remove from the oven and add the Brussels sprouts, using a metal spatula to mix them into the vegetables on the tray. Flip the sausages over and return the tray to the oven for a further 20–30 minutes until the vegetables are becoming golden and the sausages are browned.

4 Combine the dressing ingredients in a jam jar, screw on the lid and shake. Pour over the contents of the tray and serve.

VARIATION

Swap the pork sausages for frozen vegetarian sausages. As they need less time to cook, add them to the tray in the final 15 minutes of cooking, flipping them over halfway through.

JOE'S TIP

If your trays are too small to hold all of the ingredients, divide them between two medium trays instead of one big one. It's important to not crowd the vegetables too much or they won't get a chance to caramelise properly.

ROASTED GNOCCHI WITH MEATBALLS, PEPPERS & SAGE

Gnocchi is one of my favourite things to make for me and the kids now. It's so simple and really quick, and you can easily find it in most supermarkets. I use sausages to make the meatballs in this recipe because they really give the dish so much flavour and taste amazing with the sage.

SERVES 4

8 (about 350g) high-quality pork sausages, removed from their casings

1 tbsp light olive oil, plus extra for drizzling

2 x 400g tins of cherry tomatoes

400g frozen sliced peppers

1 tbsp balsamic vinegar

1 tsp dried oregano

pinch each of salt and freshly ground black pepper

500g gnocchi

12 sage leaves

Parmesan cheese, finely grated, to serve

1 Preheat the oven to 220°C/200°C fan.

2 Take heaped teaspoonfuls of the sausagemeat and roll into small meatballs. Toss the meatballs with the oil on a large rimmed baking tray or in a roasting tin. Bake for 10 minutes so they start to brown slightly.

3 Remove the tray from the oven and flip the meatballs over. Add the tinned tomatoes, peppers, balsamic vinegar and dried oregano to the tray. Sprinkle on the salt and pepper, then stir everything together. Gently shake the tray a few times to spread everything out evenly. Return to the oven for 25 minutes, stirring halfway through, until the sauce is thickened.

4 Remove the tray from the oven. Toss the gnocchi with the sage leaves and a drizzle of oil, then spread out over the tray. Return to the oven to bake for another 5 minutes to warm the gnocchi through.

5 Turn the oven to the grill setting and grill for 2–3 minutes until the meatballs and gnocchi are slightly browned on top.

6 Remove from the oven and sprinkle with some grated Parmesan before serving.

VARIATION

Use veggie sausages in place of the pork sausages. These often don't have casings, so you can just chop them into small pieces and roll into balls.

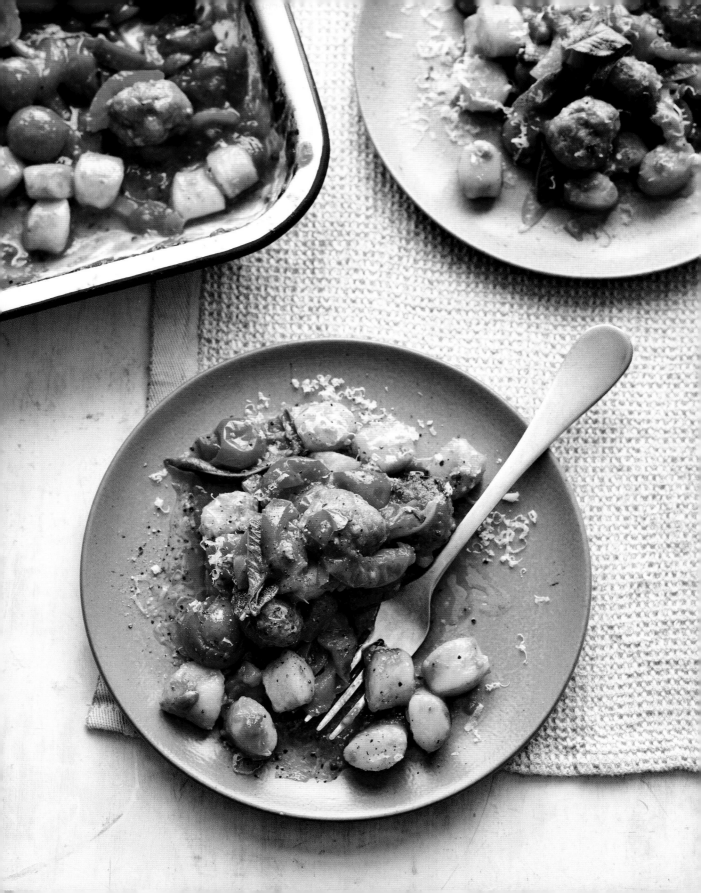

ROAST SQUASH & HALLOUMI WITH BULGUR WHEAT & CHILLI GINGER DRESSING

Roasted butternut squash tastes out of this world, and combining it with bulgur wheat means this colourful dish is packed with fibre. The pumpkin seeds give it a great crunchy texture, too. With grilled halloumi and a zingy dressing, this is a real feel good recipe.

SERVES 4

1 butternut squash, peeled, seeds removed, cut into 3cm chunks

1 tbsp light olive oil

pinch of salt

300g cherry tomatoes

200g bulgur wheat

30g fresh flat-leaf parsley, roughly chopped

30g fresh coriander, roughly chopped

100g baby spinach

4 tbsp pumpkin seeds

225g halloumi cheese, cut into 5mm-thick planks

Dressing

juice of 1 lime

1 tsp grated fresh ginger

1 garlic clove, crushed

2 tbsp extra-virgin olive oil

½ red chilli, seeds removed, finely chopped (optional)

pinch of salt

1 Preheat the oven to 200°C/180°C fan.

2 Toss the squash with the oil and the salt on a large baking tray. Roast for 20–25 minutes until starting to soften.

3 Remove the tray from the oven, flip the squash pieces over, then scatter on the cherry tomatoes. Roast for a further 20–25 minutes until the tomatoes have burst and the squash is beginning to brown.

4 Cook the bulgur wheat in a pan of boiling water for 15 minutes, then drain, return to the pan and cover with a lid. Leave to stand for 5 minutes so it can steam, then tip into a serving bowl. Stir through the chopped parsley, coriander and baby spinach.

5 Shake the dressing ingredients together in a jar until emulsified, then set aside.

6 Toast the pumpkin seeds in a medium, dry frying pan on the stove over a high heat – they're done when they start to pop and puff. Tip them into the bowl with the bulgur wheat.

7 Return the frying pan to the heat. Add the halloumi and cook until golden on both sides.

8 Divide the bulgur wheat mixture between 4 bowls and top with the roasted veg and fried halloumi. Pour over the dressing and serve.

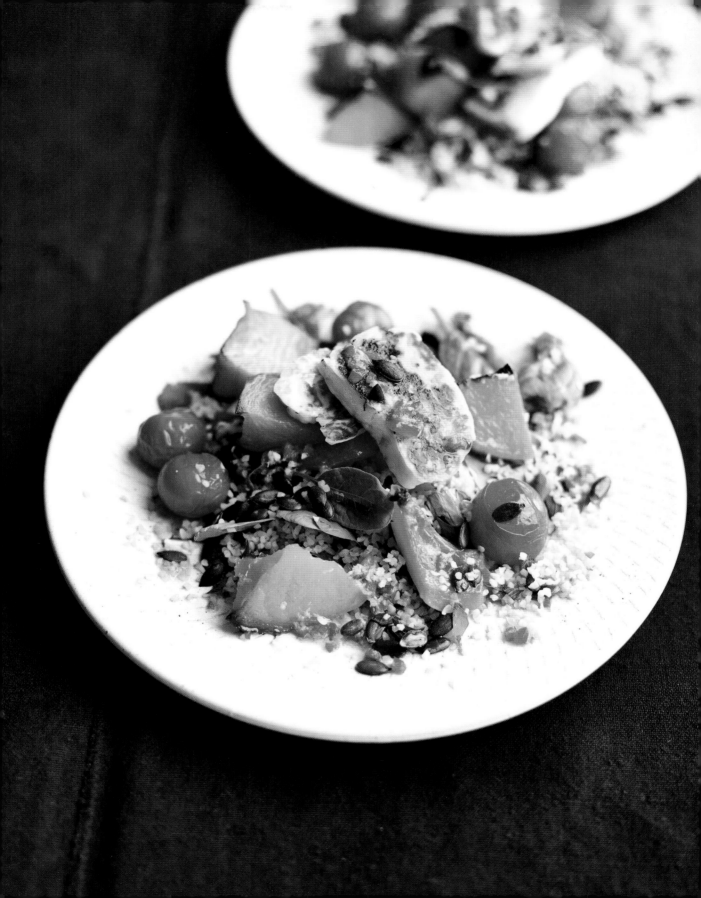

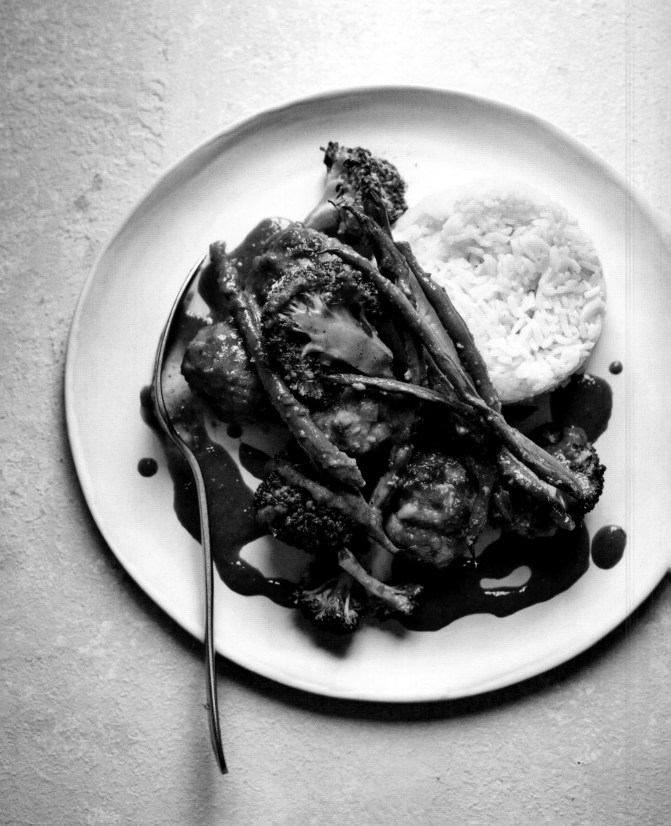

PORK SATAY MEATBALL TRAYBAKE

If you love peanut satay sauce, then this recipe will be right up your street. The pork meatballs are so soft and tender and taste incredible. I could eat this every week. I hope you love it as much as I do!

SERVES 4

1 tbsp coconut oil

1 head of broccoli, cut into small florets

500g minced pork

2 eggs

30g panko breadcrumbs

200g carrot, coarsely grated

1 small or ½ large white onion, finely diced

1 tbsp soy sauce

150g green beans, trimmed

For the Rice

180g jasmine rice

300ml water

pinch of salt

Satay Sauce

4 tbsp smooth peanut butter

4 tbsp soy sauce

2 tsp apple cider vinegar

2 tsp runny honey

2 garlic cloves, crushed

2 tsp grated fresh ginger

4 tsp sriracha, or other hot sauce

4 tsp water

1 Preheat the oven to 200°C/180°C fan.

2 Place the coconut oil on a large, rimmed baking tray and put into the oven for 1 minute to melt. Toss the broccoli onto the tray and stir to coat with the oil.

3 In a large bowl mix the pork, eggs, breadcrumbs, grated carrot, onion and soy sauce. Squish together by hand, then roll into tablespoon-sized balls. Scatter these among the broccoli on the tray. Bake for 10 minutes.

4 Meanwhile, cook the rice. Wash the rice until the water runs mostly clear. Tip into a medium saucepan, add the measured water and a pinch of salt. Bring to the boil over a high heat, then reduce the heat to low, cover with a lid and cook for 10 minutes. Remove from the heat and leave the lid on for a further 7 minutes to steam.

5 Remove the tray from the oven, add the green beans and return to the oven to a further 10 minutes.

6 Mix together all of the satay sauce ingredients in a small bowl.

7 Remove the tray from the oven and spoon a little satay sauce over the meatballs, reserving the rest for serving. Turn the oven to the grill setting and return the tray to the oven for 2–4 minutes until the meatballs are browned.

8 Serve the meatballs and veg with the cooked jasmine rice and reserved satay sauce.

BAKED TOMATO RISOTTO

Baked risotto means no more standing over the stove stirring for 30 minutes, and you still get perfectly cooked rice and a creamy texture. With just a little chorizo for its fiery flavour, this tomato risotto will blow you away. I can't wait for you to try this one.

SERVES 4

2 x 400g tins of cherry tomatoes

3 tbsp light olive oil

1 tsp dried oregano

1 chicken or vegetable stock cube

80g chorizo, diced

3 carrots, finely diced

2 celery sticks, finely diced

1 red onion, finely diced

300g risotto rice (arborio or carnaroli)

2 tbsp reduced-fat crème fraîche

salt and freshly ground black pepper

grated Parmesan, to serve

1 Preheat your oven to 220°C/200°C fan. Boil the kettle.

2 Set a sieve over a medium bowl. Empty the tins of cherry tomatoes into the sieve, catching the tomato juice in the bowl underneath. Tip the cherry tomatoes onto a rimmed baking tray, drizzle with 2 tablespoons of the oil, and sprinkle with the oregano and a pinch of salt. Roast in the oven for 25–30 minutes until starting to brown.

3 Pour the tomato juice from the bowl into a jug. Crumble in the stock cube and pour in enough boiling water to bring the level to 900ml. Set aside.

4 Place an ovenproof pot or casserole dish over a medium heat and add the diced chorizo. Cook until the fat has rendered and the chorizo is crisp. Add the remaining tablespoon of olive oil, the carrots, celery and onion, and stir to coat in the oil. Continue to cook over a medium-low heat for about 15 minutes until softened and starting to brown. Add the rice and stir for a minute so that it toasts slightly, then pour in the tomato/stock mixture, stir and bring to a simmer. Cover with a lid and bake in the oven for 15–20 minutes until the rice is just cooked.

5 Remove from the oven and take off the lid. Return to the stove over a medium heat and stir in 100–150ml hot water along with the crème fraîche. Stir until the mixture looks loose and creamy (it should form a puddle, not a mound, when scooped into a spoon). Taste and season with salt and pepper, as needed.

6 Divide between 4 bowls and top with the roasted tomatoes and a grating of Parmesan.

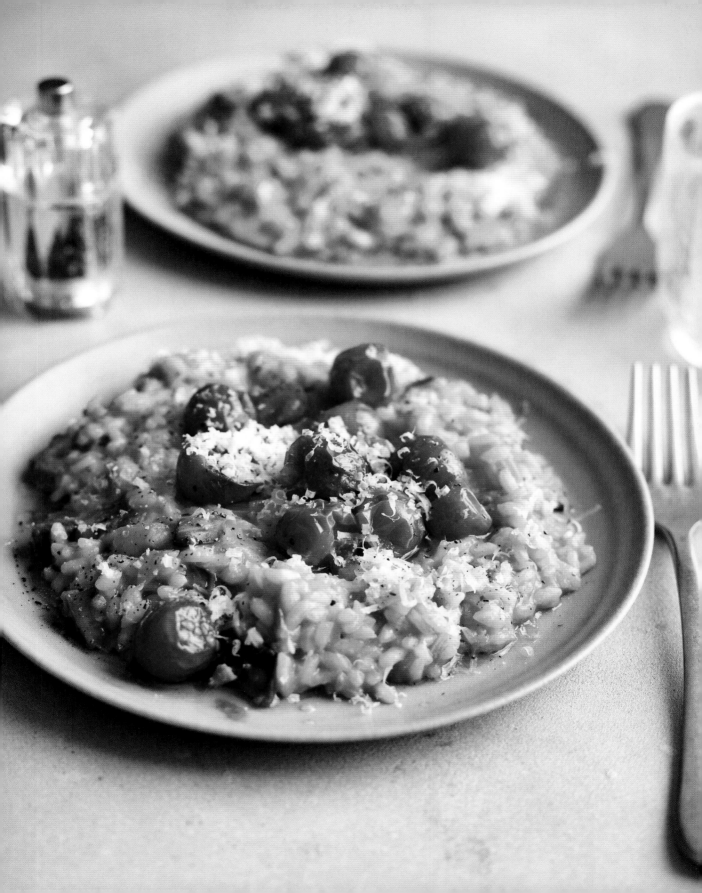

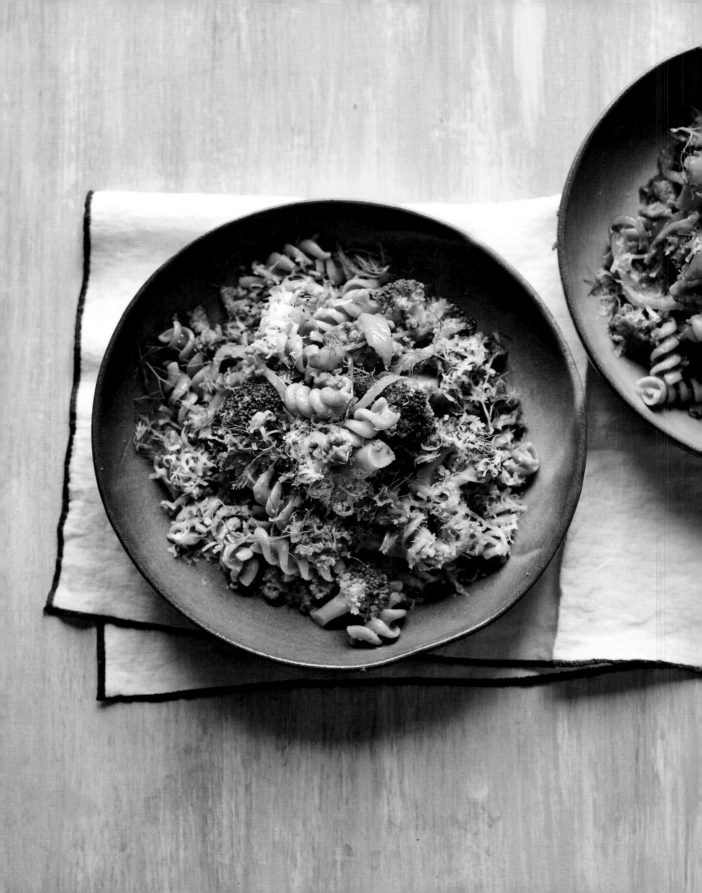

SAUSAGE, FENNEL & BROCCOLI PASTA

Another absolute belter of a pasta dish. You will love this one, I'm sure. I think sausage and fennel is one of the best combinations ever. The sausagemeat just has so much flavour, so get some decent ones in there. This recipe will also work with any type of pasta, so mix it up if you fancy it with spaghetti, penne or even gnocchi.

SERVES 4

1 head of broccoli, cut into small florets

300g wholemeal fusilli pasta

2 tbsp light olive oil

1 bulb of fennel, thinly sliced

400g high-quality pork sausages, casings removed

2 garlic cloves, crushed

½ tsp chilli flakes

juice of ½ lemon

salt, to taste

25g Parmesan cheese, finely grated, to serve

1 Bring a large pan of water to the boil and add the broccoli. Cook for 10 minutes until very soft, then use a slotted spoon to remove the broccoli to a bowl.

2 Add the pasta to the pan and cook according to the packet instructions. Drain the pasta, reserving some of the pasta water, and set aside.

3 Meanwhile, heat the olive oil in a large frying pan over a medium heat. Add the fennel and a pinch of salt, then cover the pan with a lid. Cook for 15 minutes, removing the lid to stir occasionally, until the fennel has softened and is golden.

4 Add the sausagemeat to the frying pan and cook until browned. Stir in the crushed garlic and chilli flakes for 1 minute, then add the cooked broccoli and pasta along with a splash of the pasta cooking water and the lemon juice. Stir together until combined, then taste and season with salt, as needed.

5 Serve, sprinkled with Parmesan.

JOE'S TIPS

- If you can't get a fennel bulb, use 1 tbsp fennel seeds instead, sautéing them in the olive oil for only 1–2 minutes until fragrant, before adding the sausagemeat.
- If you are serving this to kids who are fussy about green veg, break down the broccoli into a kind of pesto when you stir it into the sausagemeat mix – they'll hardly notice it.

CREAMY COURGETTE & BASIL PASTA

Pasta is life. I love the stuff. Any shape, any size, any sauce. This one has a really yummy, creamy veg-packed sauce with a beautiful fresh basil pesto. Eat this hot or cold, just be sure to give it a nice generous sprinkle of cheese on top for the win.

SERVES 4

4 tbsp light olive oil

20g dried breadcrumbs

¼ tsp dried oregano

finely grated zest and juice of ½ lemon

30g vegetarian hard cheese or Parmesan, finely grated, plus extra to serve

4 medium courgettes, cut into 4cm chunks

4 garlic cloves, crushed

350g wholemeal penne pasta (or another short pasta shape)

30g fresh basil leaves

salt

simple salad, to serve

1 Heat 1 tablespoon of the olive oil in a large frying pan over a high heat. Once hot, add the breadcrumbs, stirring to coat them with the oil. Toast, stirring constantly, until they are uniformly golden. Tip them into a small bowl and mix in a pinch of salt, the dried oregano, lemon zest and a third of the grated cheese. Set aside.

2 Return the pan to a medium-low heat, add the remaining 3 tablespoons of oil, the courgettes and a pinch of salt. Cook for about 15 minutes, stirring occasionally, until soft and caramelised. Stir in the garlic and cook for 1 minute, then remove from the heat.

3 Meanwhile, cook the pasta in a large pan of well-salted water, according to the packet instructions. Drain, reserving some of the pasta cooking water, and return the pasta to the pan.

4 Take half of the cooked courgettes from the pan and blitz them with the lemon juice, remaining cheese and basil leaves until smooth (you can use a food processor, blender or hand blender). Pour this sauce into the pan of cooked pasta and stir through. If the sauce is a bit thick, loosen with some of the pasta cooking water. Taste and season with salt, as needed.

5 Divide between 4 bowls and top with the remaining courgettes and toasted breadcrumbs. Serve with a salad, with extra grated cheese on the side for everyone to help themsleves.

JOE'S TIPS

- **Swapping white pasta to wholemeal is such an easy, healthy switch-up. Wholemeal pasta is much higher in fibre, which contributes to your digestive health and general wellbeing.**
- **Cooking and blitzing the courgettes means you get a really creamy texture to this sauce. If you are serving this to kids who are fussy about chunks of veg, just blitz the whole lot.**

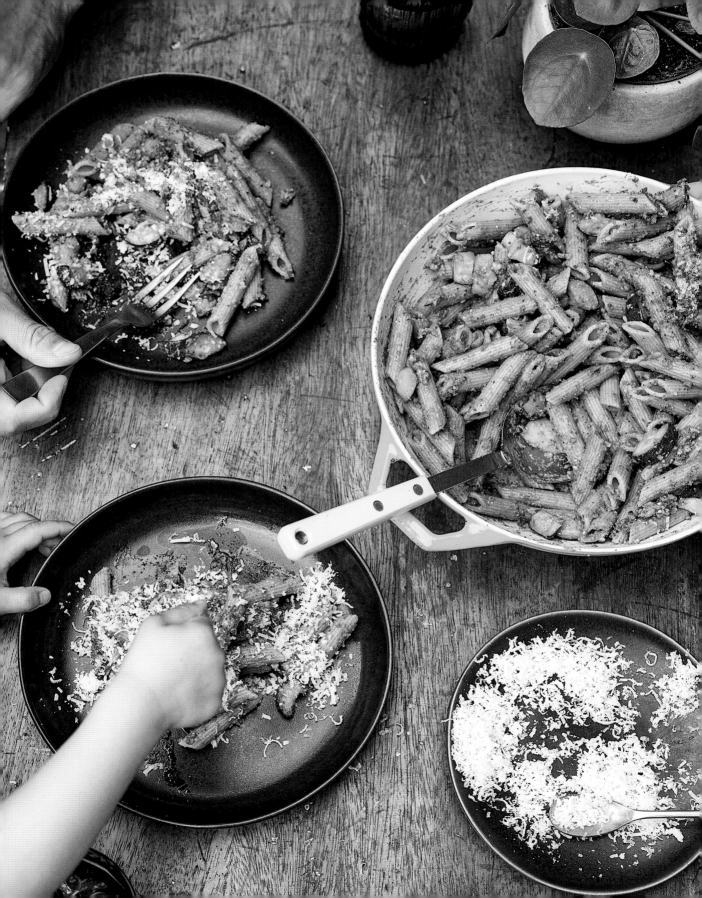

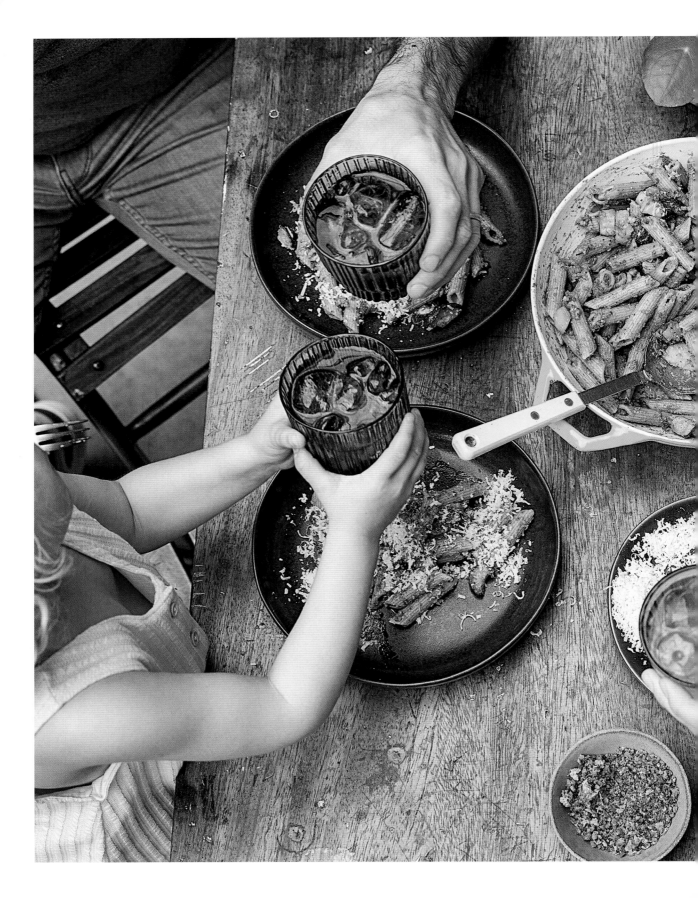

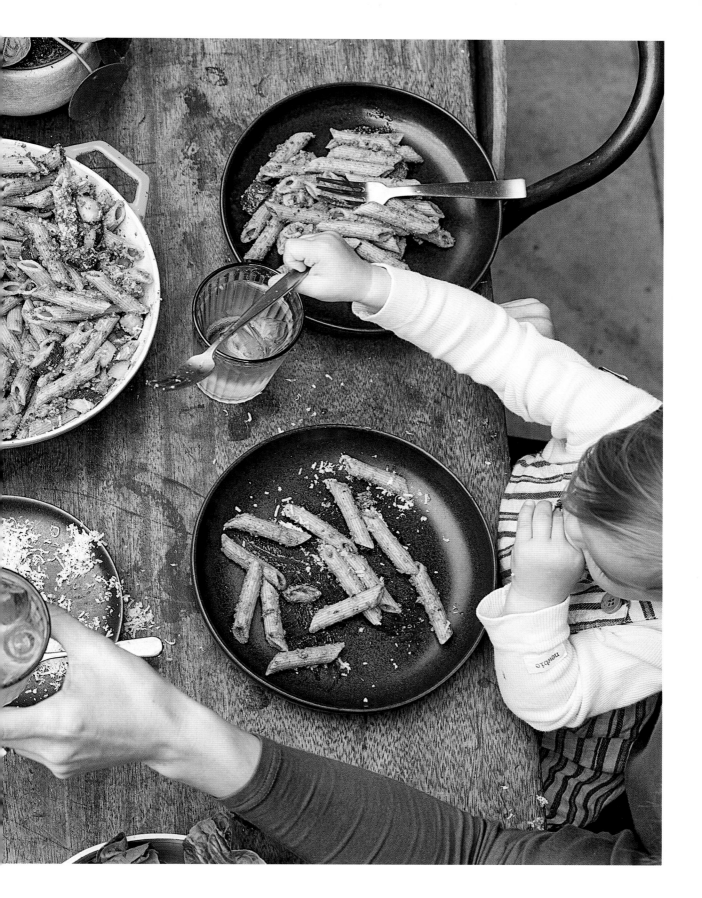

CREAMY KALE, COURGETTE & BUTTER BEAN TORTELLINI PASTA BAKE

Pasta bakes have become a weekly favourite in my house. I love how hassle-free they are to just knock together and leave in the oven for a while. This recipe uses store-bought stuffed pasta but combines it with lots of healthy and nutritious vegetables.

SERVES 4

1 tbsp light olive oil

2 courgettes, cut into 3cm chunks

2 garlic cloves, crushed

200g kale, chopped

2 x 300g packs of ready-made ricotta-and-spinach-stuffed tortellini or tortelloni pasta

400g tin of butter beans, drained and rinsed

4 tbsp breadcrumbs (fresh or dried)

Cheese Sauce

2 tbsp extra-virgin olive oil

4 tbsp plain white flour

400ml semi-skimmed milk

250ml water

2 tsp Dijon mustard

2 tsp lemon juice

1 low-salt vegetable stock cube

70g mature Cheddar cheese, grated

salt and freshly ground black pepper

1 First, make the cheese sauce. Heat the extra-virgin olive oil in a medium saucepan over a medium heat, add the flour and stir to combine. Cook for 1–2 minutes to lightly toast the flour, then gradually whisk in the milk until smooth. Stir in the water, mustard and lemon juice, and crumble in the stock cube, and cook, stirring occasionally, until thickened. Mix in the grated cheese, season with salt and pepper to taste, and remove from the heat.

2 In a large, non-stick frying pan, heat the light olive oil over a medium heat. Add the courgette chunks and cook, stirring occasionally, until golden all over. Stir in the garlic and cook for 1 minute, then remove from the heat.

3 Preheat the grill to high.

4 Bring a large pan of water to the boil. Once boiling, add the chopped kale and the tortellini. Cook for 2–3 minutes (or according to the pasta packet instructions), then drain and return to the pan.

5 Stir the cheese sauce, sautéed courgettes and drained butter beans into the pan, then tip the whole mixture into a 23 x 33cm (or a similar size) baking dish. Sprinkle with the breadcrumbs and place under the grill for 4–6 minutes or until bubbling and golden on top.

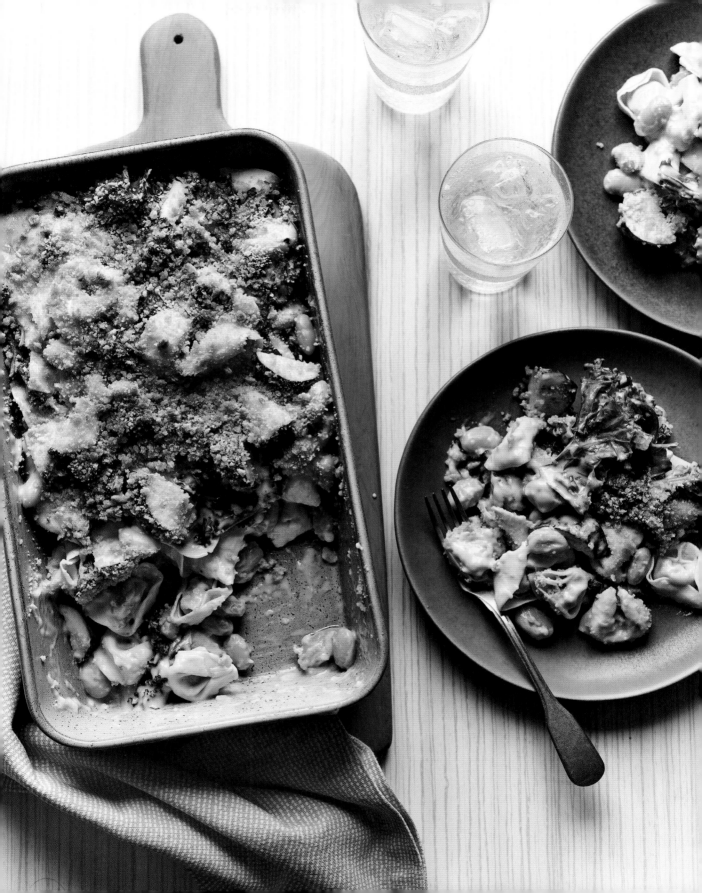

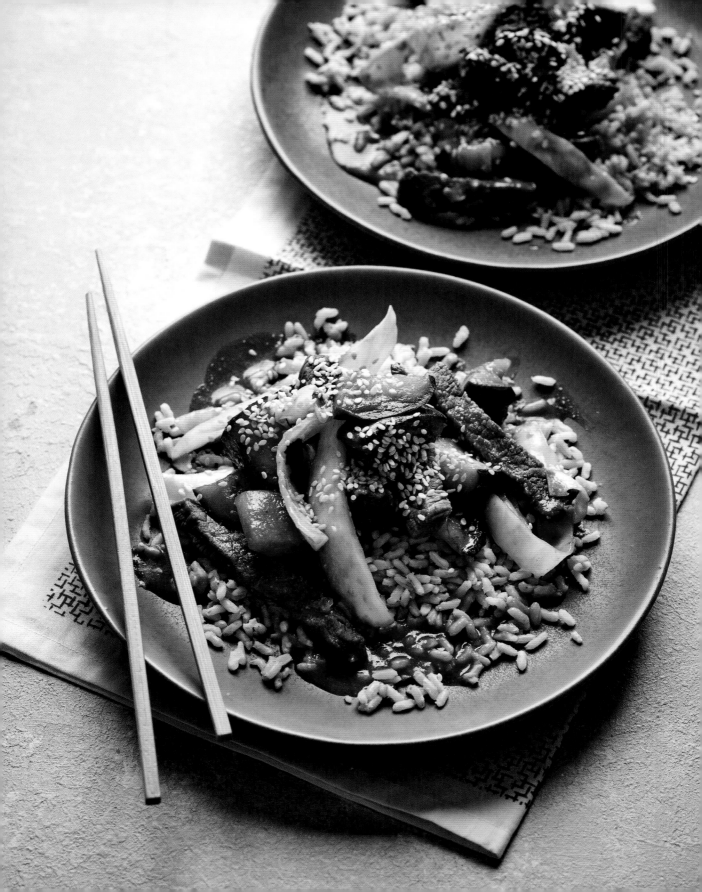

JAPANESE-STYLE BEEF, AUBERGINE & MISO STIR-FRY

This is a super-tasty, sticky stir-fry, that's packed full of the good stuff. The number one rule when stir-frying is to always make sure you have everything chopped and ready to go, then it can be cooked in a flash. Serve with brown or white rice and a sprinkling of sesame seeds.

SERVES 4

2 aubergines, cut into 3cm chunks

pinch of salt

2 tbsp cornflour

1–2 tbsp light olive oil

¼ head of cabbage, cut into 2cm-wide ribbons

350g beef stir-fry strips

Miso Sauce

2 tbsp white miso paste

2 tbsp mirin or Marsala/sherry

1 tbsp soy sauce (low-sodium, if possible)

2 tsp honey

150ml water

To Serve

500g cooked brown or white rice

1 tbsp sesame seeds

1 Sprinkle the aubergine chunks with a pinch of salt and set aside in a colander for 10 minutes. Rinse the aubergines to remove the salt, then squeeze to remove any excess liquid. Add to a large bowl with the cornflour and toss to coat.

2 Heat 1 tablespoon of the oil in a large, non-stick frying pan over a medium heat. Add half of the aubergine chunks and cook until starting to brown. Remove to a plate, then cook the remaining aubergine in the same way, adding another tablespoon of oil to the pan, if needed. Remove to the plate.

3 Return the pan to the heat, add the cabbage and stir-fry over a high heat until starting to brown. Remove to the same plate as the aubergine.

4 Return the pan to the heat, add the beef strips and stir-fry over a high heat until browned, then stir in the garlic for 1 minute.

5 Mix together the miso sauce ingredients in a small bowl until smooth, then pour into the pan along with the aubergine and cabbage. Cook, stirring occasionally, until the sauce has thickened slightly, around 5 minutes.

6 Serve the stir-fry with cooked rice and a sprinkle of sesame seeds.

JOE'S TIP

If you don't have mirin or Marsala/sherry, you can replace it with 2 tsp lemon juice plus 1 tsp honey, instead.

GRILLED SALMON WITH SPICY CORN & PINEAPPLE SALSA

This is the ultimate feel good recipe, with omega-3 fatty acids from the salmon and fibre from the wholegrain rice. The spicy corn and pineapple salsa is really worth the effort, too. I think you will love this one. Enjoy!

SERVES 4

1 tbsp sriracha, or other hot sauce

1½ tsp maple syrup

1 tsp apple cider vinegar

½ tsp ground cumin

4 x 150g skin-on salmon fillets

400g sugar snap peas

300g cooked brown rice, to serve

Spicy Corn and Pineapple Salsa

1 regular or 2 mini corn cobs

1 tomato, diced

100g pineapple, finely chopped

juice of ½ lime

handful of fresh coriander

½ jalapeño, diced

pinch of salt

1 Start with the salsa. Preheat a griddle pan over a high heat. Once hot, add the corn and grill, turning occasionally, until charred. Let the corn cool slightly, then use a sharp knife to cut the kernels from the cob.

2 Add the charred corn to a medium bowl with the tomato, pineapple, lime juice, coriander, jalapeño and salt. Stir together and set aside.

3 Mix the sriracha, maple syrup, apple cider vinegar and cumin in a small bowl. Set aside.

4 Add the salmon fillets to the griddle pan, skin-side down. Cook for 4–5 minutes until the skin is crispy, then flip and cook on the other side for 2–3 minutes until cooked through. Remove from the pan and drizzle with the sriracha mixture.

5 Add the sugar snap peas to the griddle pan and cook until slightly charred.

6 Serve the grilled salmon with the salsa, charred sugar snaps and cooked brown rice.

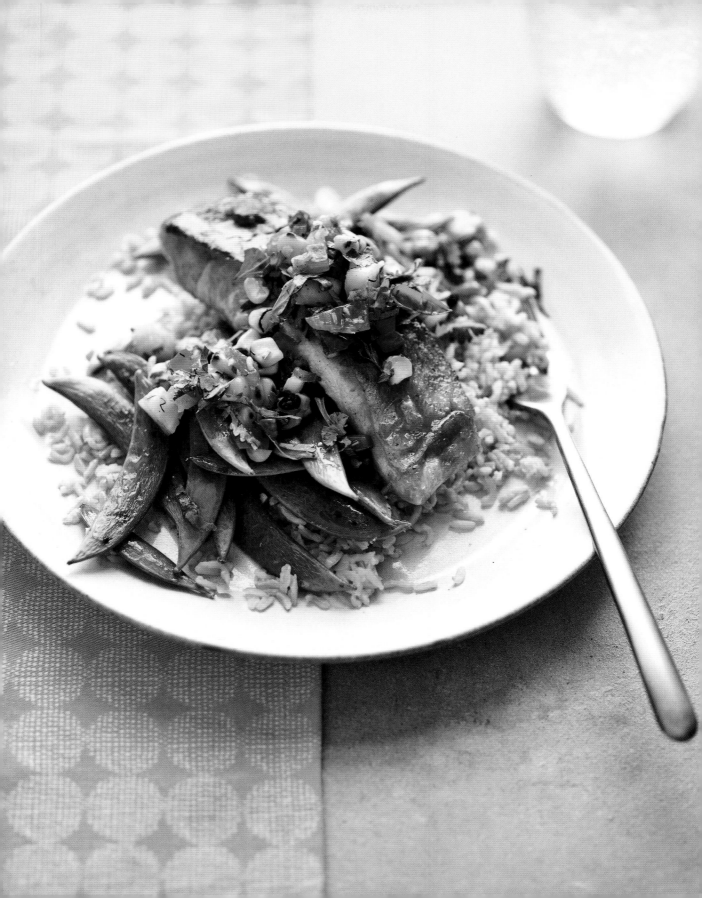

BLACK-BEAN BEEF, BASIL & PEANUT STIR-FRY

A classic Chinese-style stir-fry, which is healthy and tastes even better than a takeaway. I think you'll be making it over and over again. The peanuts are great for an extra crunch and add more flavour, but feel free to leave them out if you want to.

SERVES 4

2 tbsp light olive oil

1 large or 2 small red onions, cut into quarters, layers separated

200g green beans, trimmed

175g baby corn, cut into 2cm chunks

250g beef stir-fry strips

1 tbsp cornflour

4 garlic cloves, crushed

1 tbsp grated ginger

250ml beef stock

100g black bean stir-fry sauce

250g medium egg noodles

handful of fresh Thai basil leaves

handful of salted peanuts, roughly chopped

1 Heat 1 tablespoon of the olive oil in a wok or large, non-stick frying pan over a high heat. Once hot, add the onions, beans and baby corn. Cook over a high heat, stirring often, until browned and softened. Remove to a plate and set aside.

2 Toss the beef strips with the cornflour. Add the remaining tablespoon of oil to the wok or frying pan and, once hot, add the beef. Stir often until browned, then mix in the garlic and ginger and stir for 1 minute more. Reduce the heat to medium-low and add the beef stock, black bean sauce and the cooked vegetables. Cook until the sauce has thickened slightly, then remove from the heat.

3 Bring a large pan of water to the boil and cook the egg noodles according to the packet instructions.

4 Drain the noodles and divide between 4 bowls, then top with the beef mixture. Garnish with the basil leaves and peanuts, then serve.

FEEL GOOD FACT

This is rich in iron and vitamin B12 from the beef, and fibre from the baby corn and green beans. Carbs are supplied by the egg noodles, which are super-quick to cook and are perfect for speedy dinners. The flavoursome black bean sauce contains no saturated fats, so is a heart-healthy addition.

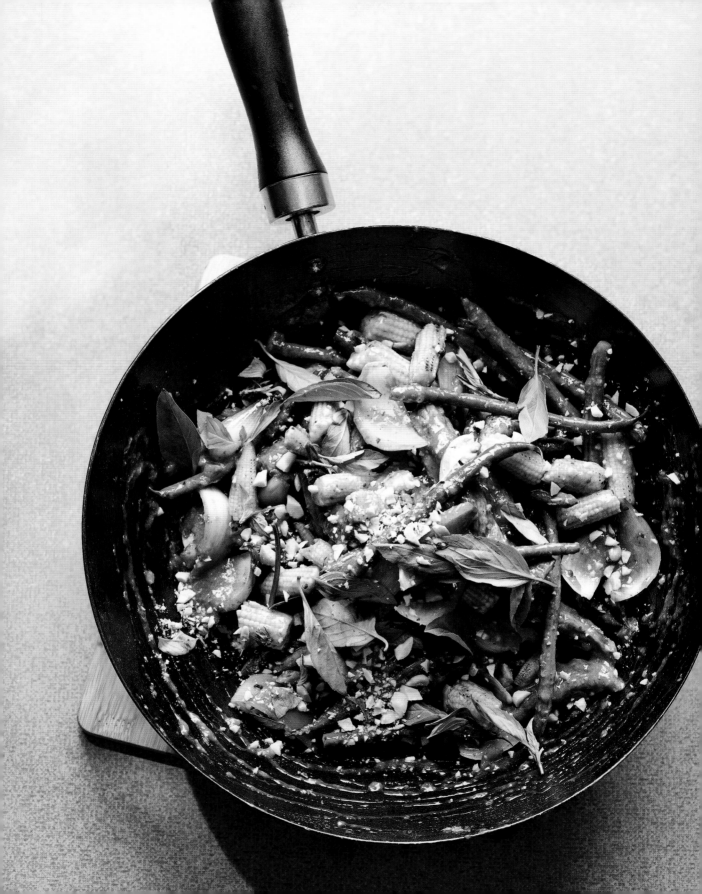

BLACK PEPPER
PRAWN NOODLES

This hot, peppery stir-fry will really liven up your tastebuds! Stir-fries are such a great way of getting loads of nutritious, vibrant ingredients with lots of colour into one bowl. The real win, though, is their speed and simplicity. Udon noodles are very quick to cook, so are great to use, but feel free to use egg noodles or rice noodles, if you prefer (see Tips).

SERVES 4

1 tbsp light olive oil

1 tsp toasted sesame oil

4 garlic cloves, crushed

1 tsp grated fresh ginger

½ head of cabbage, cut into 1cm-wide ribbons

2 carrots, coarsely grated

1 red bell pepper, seeds removed and thinly sliced

200g sugar snap peas

2 tbsp oyster sauce

2 tbsp soy sauce

1 tbsp Shaoxing rice wine

2 tsp freshly ground black pepper

½ tsp ground white pepper

600g fresh udon noodles

200g frozen cooked prawns, defrosted

4 spring onions, thinly sliced

1 Heat the olive oil and sesame oil in a large wok or a large frying pan over a high heat. Add the garlic and ginger and stir for a minute before adding the cabbage, carrots, bell pepper and sugar snap peas. Cook, stirring often, until the vegetables have softened slightly and are starting to brown.

2 Add the oyster sauce, soy sauce, rice wine, black and white pepper, stirring to coat the vegetables, then add the udon noodles. Stir them in a bit so they're covered with a layer of vegetables, then cover the pan with a lid (or a baking tray). Reduce the heat to low and cook for 4 minutes to soften the noodles.

3 Remove the lid and gently separate the noodles, then stir in the defrosted, cooked prawns to warm through.

4 Divide between 4 plates and serve garnished with the spring onions.

JOE'S TIPS

- Different varieties of fresh noodles can be added at the same point in step 2 that the udon noodles are added.
- If you want to swap in your own choice of dried noodles, cook them first according to the packet instructions and add them to the pan with the prawns in step 3.

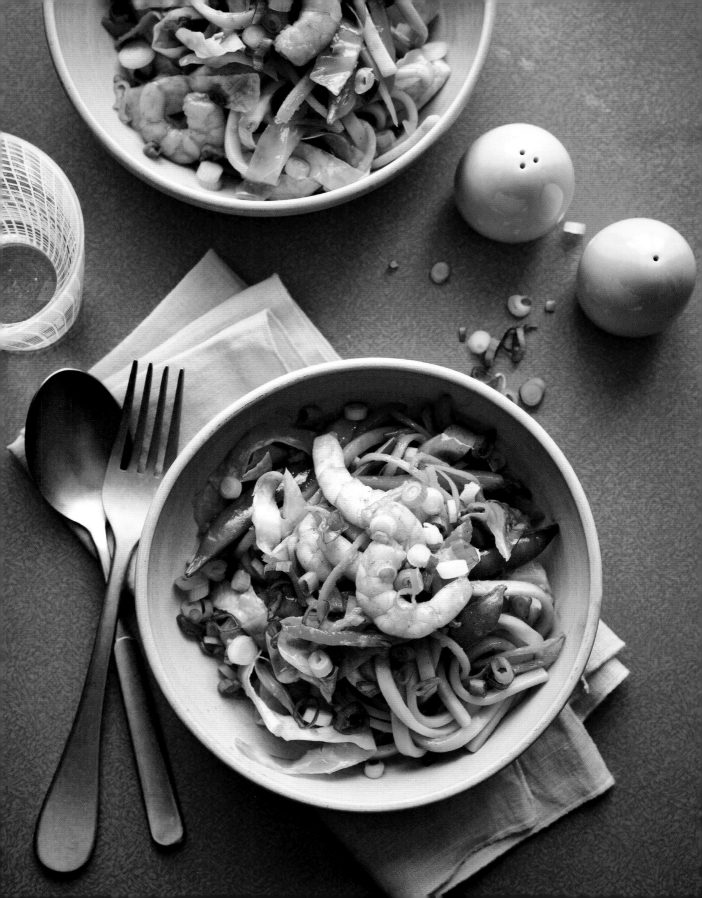

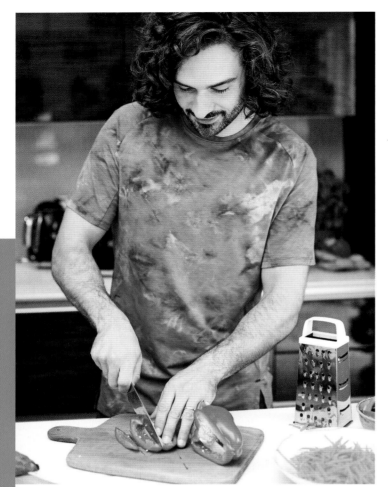
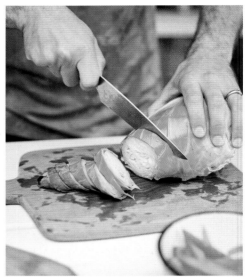
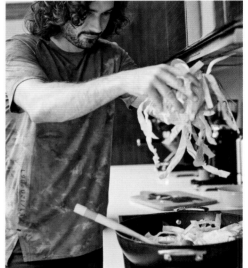
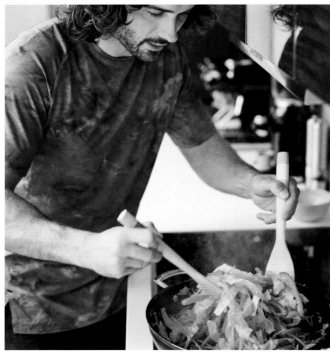
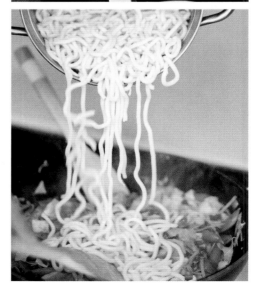

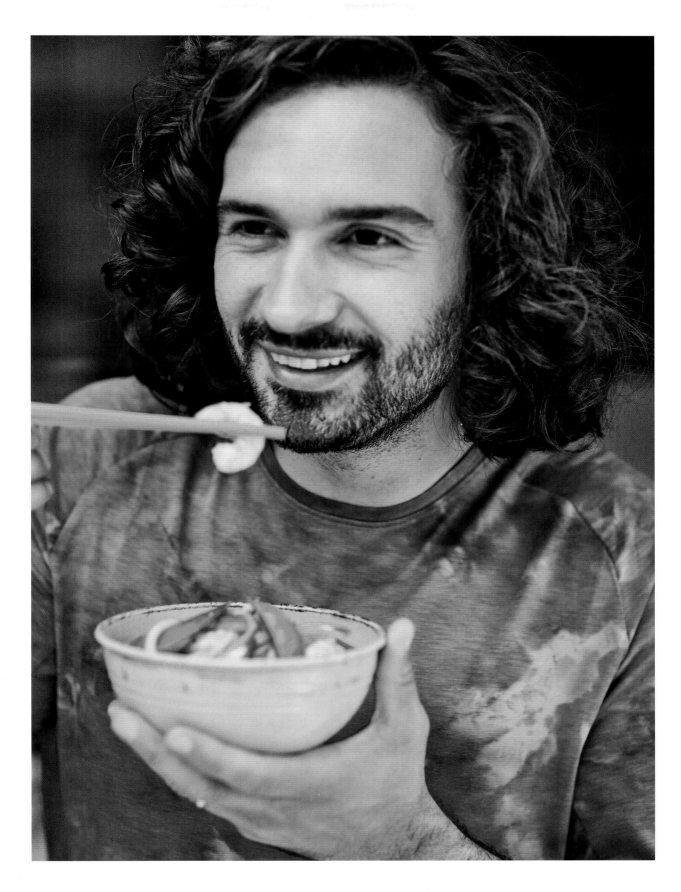

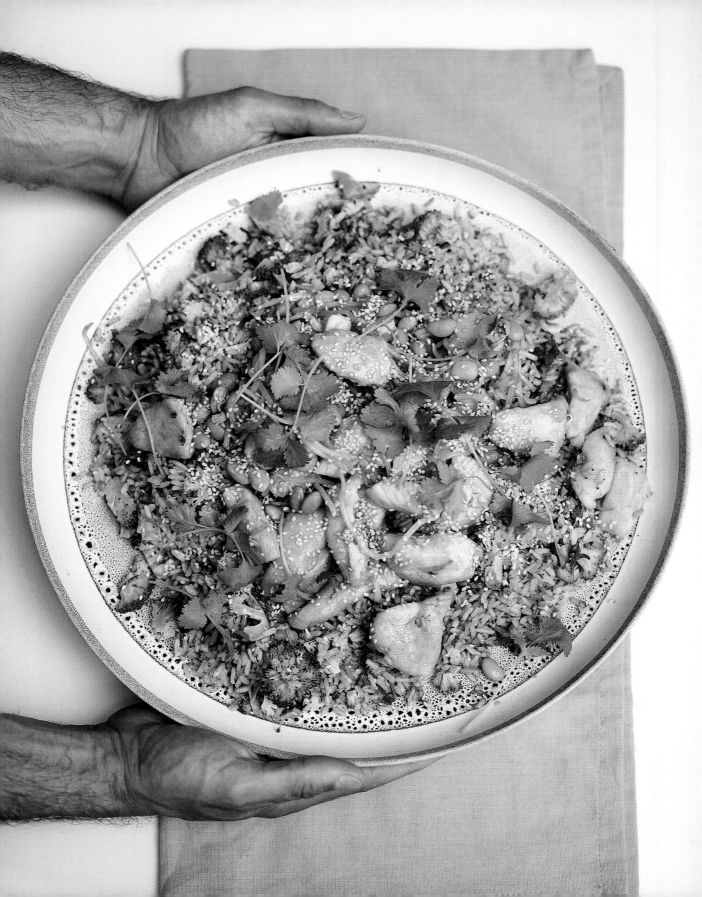

SESAME CHICKEN STIR-FRY WITH BROCCOLI RICE

This is one of my favourite stir-fry recipes. I make this a lot because it's so quick to cook and the kids love it, too. The home-made sesame sauce just tastes wicked with the fried chicken and crunchy broccoli. Great for a family meal or a get-together with friends.

SERVES 4

1 large head of broccoli

3 chicken breasts, cut into bite-sized pieces

1½ tbsp cornflour

1 tbsp refined coconut oil or light olive oil

75g frozen podded edamame beans

100g beansprouts

1 tsp sesame oil

500g cooked brown rice

handful of fresh coriander, roughly chopped, plus extra to serve

2 tbsp toasted sesame seeds, to serve

Sesame Sauce

2 tbsp soy sauce

2 tbsp honey

1 tbsp sriracha, or other hot sauce

1 tbsp apple cider vinegar

2 tsp sesame oil

1 tbsp grated fresh ginger

1 Slice the broccoli very finely, shredding it into rice-like pieces. Set aside.

2 Toss the chicken pieces with the cornflour in a medium bowl.

3 Heat the coconut or olive oil in a large, non-stick frying pan over a high heat. Add the chicken pieces and cook, stirring, until no longer pink.

4 Mix together all of the sesame sauce ingredients in a small bowl, then pour into the chicken pan along with the edamame and beansprouts. Stir over a medium heat until the sauce has thickened slightly, then tip out into a bowl, or set aside.

5 If using the same pan, return it to the heat; alternatively, heat a separate pan over a medium heat. Add the sesame oil and the 'riced' broccoli and stir until softened. Stir in the cooked rice, then remove from the heat and fold in the coriander.

6 Serve the rice topped with the chicken and a sprinkle of sesame seeds and coriander.

CREAMY HARICOT BEANS WITH PARSLEY PESTO

Did you know that baked beans are actually made using haricot beans? When you cook haricot beans in the liquid from the tin they become extremely creamy and taste amazing. This makes a really delicious quick lunch or dinner. The fresh parsley pesto lights this one up big time, too. Something different and new for you maybe, but totally worth a try! Serve with some crusty bread and a little salad on the side.

SERVES 4

2 tbsp extra-virgin olive oil

6 sprigs of fresh thyme

6 garlic cloves, crushed

2 x 400g tins of haricot beans

1 bay leaf

1 low-salt vegetable stock cube
   (or chicken if not vegetarian)

salt and freshly ground black pepper

Parsley Pesto

20g (big handful) flat-leaf parsley leaves

10g (small handful) chives

juice of ½ lemon

2 tbsp extra-virgin olive oil

1 tbsp water

pinch of salt

To Serve

grated vegetarian hard cheese
   or Parmesan

crusty wholemeal bread rolls

simple side salad

1 Heat the oil in a medium saucepan over a medium heat. Once hot, add the thyme sprigs and sizzle for 30 seconds, then add the crushed garlic. Cook until the garlic starts to turn golden in places, then tip in the tins of beans (and their liquid) and add the bay leaf. Fill one of the tins with water and add that too, then crumble in the stock cube and season with some black pepper. Simmer for 20–30 minutes until the beans are slightly softened.

2 Remove the bay leaf and thyme sprigs. Use a stick blender to blitz about a quarter of the beans, which will make the sauce super creamy. Alternatively, use a potato masher to mash some of the beans. Taste and season with salt, if needed.

3 Make the parsley pesto by blitzing all the pesto ingredients into a paste. You can do this with a hand blender in a jug or in a food processor or blender.

4 Dish up the warm beans, drizzle with some pesto and grate over some Parmesan cheese. Serve with crusty bread for dipping and a simple salad on the side.

JOE'S TIPS

- Turn into a hearty cauliflower soup by adding ½ head of cauliflower, cut into small florets, for the final 8 minutes of cooking.
- Use other beans instead, such as cannellini, butter beans or borlotti.
- Switch up the herbs in the pesto to use up whatever soft herbs you have to hand.
- Use jarred pesto instead of making your own.
- For a quick creamy pasta sauce, stir the garlicky beans through cooked pasta and garnish with shaved Parmesan.

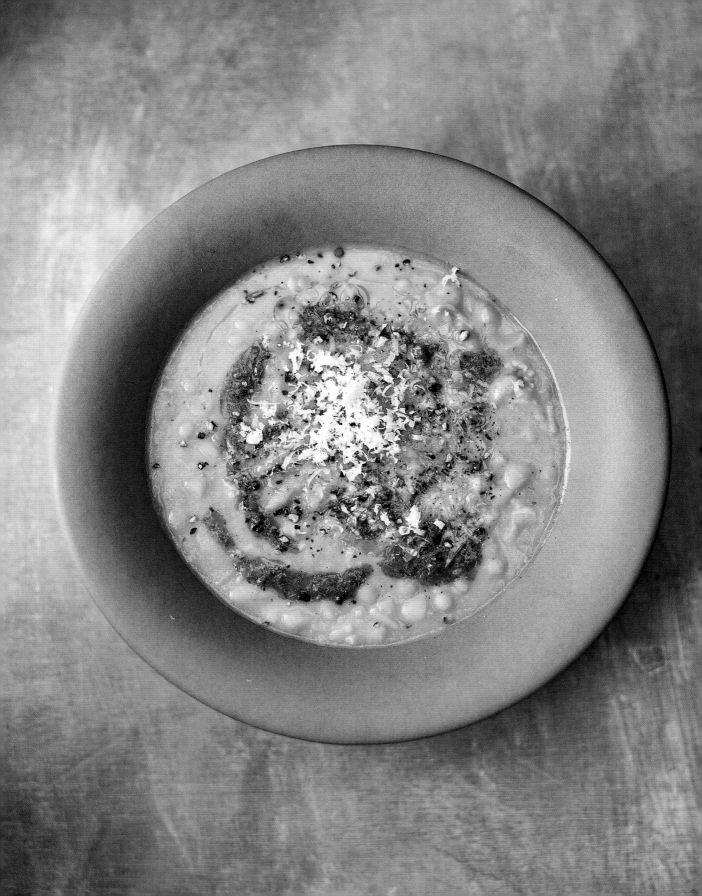

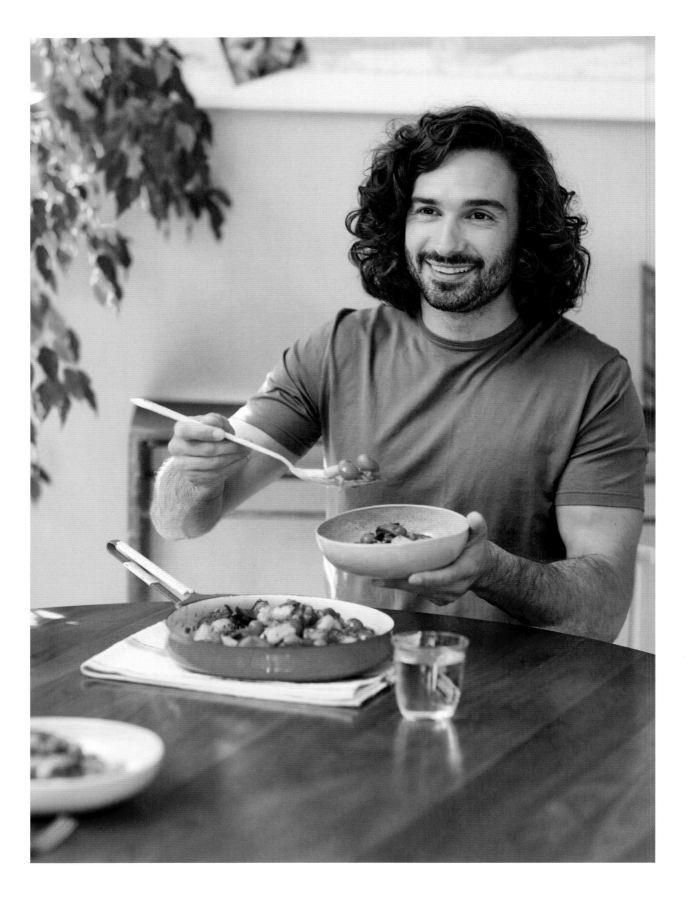

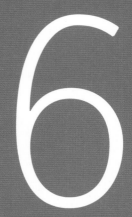

HEARTY

mains with less meat and more veg

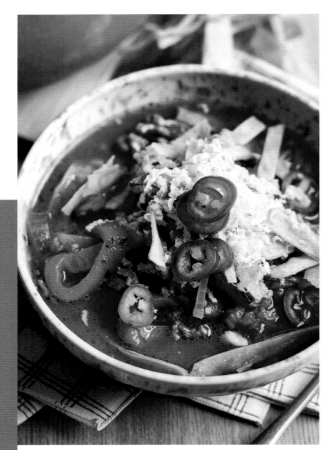

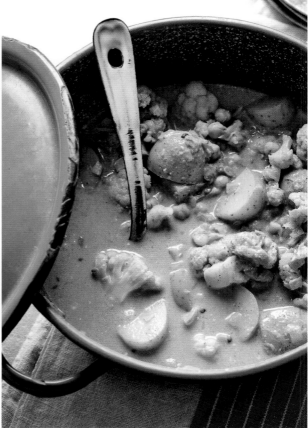

I just love all the recipes in this chapter. They make me feel all warm inside! This is the chapter to turn to when you're looking for something really substantial. Wholesome and hearty, these stews and soups will fill you up and keep you going for a long time. There are hotpots and some more sticky traybakes, too.

I don't know about you, but I often associate hearty meals with root veg and also with warming spices. With that in mind, I've got a fair few curries and chillies here, all with substantial veg content. We should all be cutting down on how much meat we eat, both for our health and for the planet, so bulking up meals with loads of veg is a great way to go.

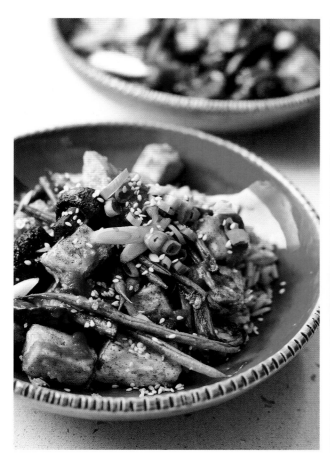

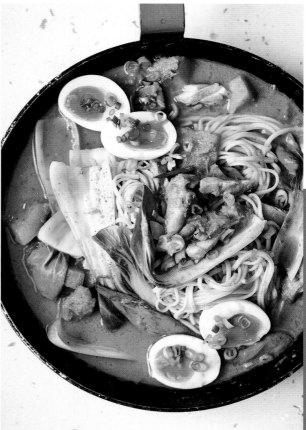

There are loads of Mediterreanean-style classics here. Believe it or not, the sun doesn't always shine in the Med, and when it's cold they have some great dishes to tuck into, such as the Spanish-style Smoky Cod, Tomato and Pepper Stew (page 229), a Bolognese with a difference (page 226) or the Chicken Orzo and Butter Bean Stew (page 206).

There are plenty of Asian flavours in this chapter too. I go mad for the Chicken and Squash Curry Ramen on page 224. It's so packed with flavour - I hope you'll love it as much as I do. And you've got to try the sticky Roasted Tofu on page 218 – what a taste sensation.

CHICKEN, ORZO & BUTTER BEAN STEW WITH PESTO

Orzo pasta always goes down well with my kids. This wholesome stew is full of flavour and great any night of the week. The chicken stock provides the rich flavour, meaning you don't have to add as much meat, and the creamy butter beans also help to bulk it out. The herby pesto provides a little zing to top it off.

SERVES 4

2 tbsp light olive oil

2 medium carrots, finely diced

3 celery sticks, finely diced

1 onion, finely diced

1 head of garlic, cloves separated

3 sprigs of thyme

2 bay leaves

750ml chicken stock

2 skinless, boneless chicken breasts

100g orzo pasta

400g tin of butter beans, drained

1–2 tbsp light soy sauce

100g cavolo nero, roughly chopped

freshly ground black pepper

Parsley and Dill Pesto

30g fresh flat-leaf parsley

20g fresh dill

4 tbsp extra-virgin olive oil

juice of 1 lemon

20g sunflower seeds, pumpkin seeds, cashews or almonds

salt

1 Heat the oil in a large saucepan over a medium-low heat, add the carrots, celery and onion and cook for about 10 minutes, stirring occasionally, until softened.

2 Gently crush each garlic clove with the side of a knife to loosen the papery casing. Place them in a medium-sized lidded jar or tupperware and put the lid on. Shake for 30 seconds, then open the lid and tip out the contents. The cloves should be peeled and you can pick out the papery casings. Roughly chop the garlic and add to the pan along with the thyme sprigs and bay leaves. Sauté for 5 minutes, stirring occasionally.

3 Pour in the chicken stock and bring to the boil, then cover and simmer for 30 minutes.

4 Add the chicken breasts, orzo and butter beans to the pan and cook for 15–20 minutes until the chicken is cooked through.

5 Remove the chicken to a cutting board and shred using two forks into bite-sized pieces. Stir the shredded chicken back into the pan along with the soy sauce (start with 1 tablespoon and taste, adding more if it needs the extra salt), cavolo nero and a good few grindings of black pepper. Cook for a couple of minutes more to wilt the cavolo nero.

6 Combine all the pesto ingredients except the salt in a food processor or blender (or in a jug, if using a hand blender) and blitz to a coarse paste. Season with salt, to taste, and thin with a bit of water to form a drizzling consistency.

7 Divide the soup between 4 bowls and top each with a spoonful of pesto.

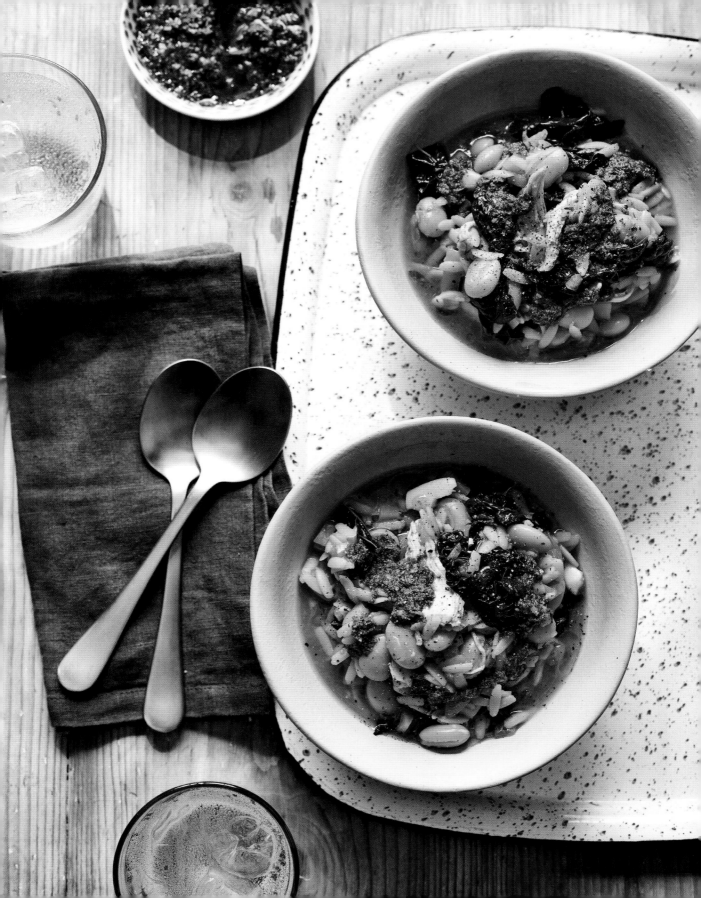

LENTIL & SUN-DRIED TOMATO PESTO SOUP

This is a really wholesome and nutritious soup. It's perfect any day of the week. Using a ready-made sun-dried tomato pesto is a quick and easy way to get a proper rich tomato flavour into your soup without the need to cook it for a long time. You will want to make this over and over again.

SERVES 4

2 tbsp light olive oil

3 medium carrots, diced

3 celery sticks, diced

2 leeks, cleaned and cut into 2cm-wide pieces

4 tbsp sun-dried tomato pesto

70g tomato purée concentrate (tomato paste)

1 litre water

1 low-salt vegetable stock cube (or chicken if not vegetarian)

2 x 250g pouches of cooked Puy lentils or 2 x 400g tins of cooked green lentils, drained and rinsed

¼ head cabbage, cut into 2cm-wide ribbons

30g vegetarian hard cheese or Parmesan, finely grated

4 lemon wedges, to serve

1 Heat the oil in a large saucepan over a medium-low heat, add the carrots, celery and leeks, and cook for about 15 minutes, stirring occasionally, until softened.

2 Add the tomato pesto and tomato purée and cook until slightly darkened, about 2 minutes, then pour in the water, crumble in the stock cube and stir in the lentils. Bring to the boil, then reduce to a simmer and cook for 15 minutes for the flavours to develop.

3 Stir in the sliced cabbage and cook for a final 5 minutes until tender.

4 Divide between 4 bowls, top with the Parmesan and serve with lemon wedges on the side.

FEEL GOOD FACT

Tomatoes are full of lycopene, an antioxidant that may be beneficial for cardiovascular health.

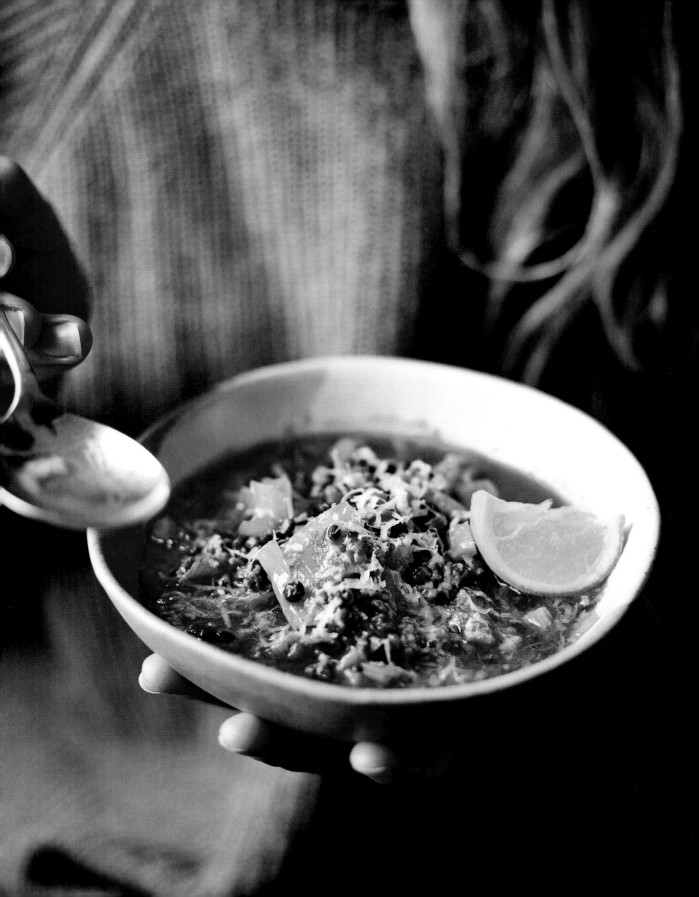

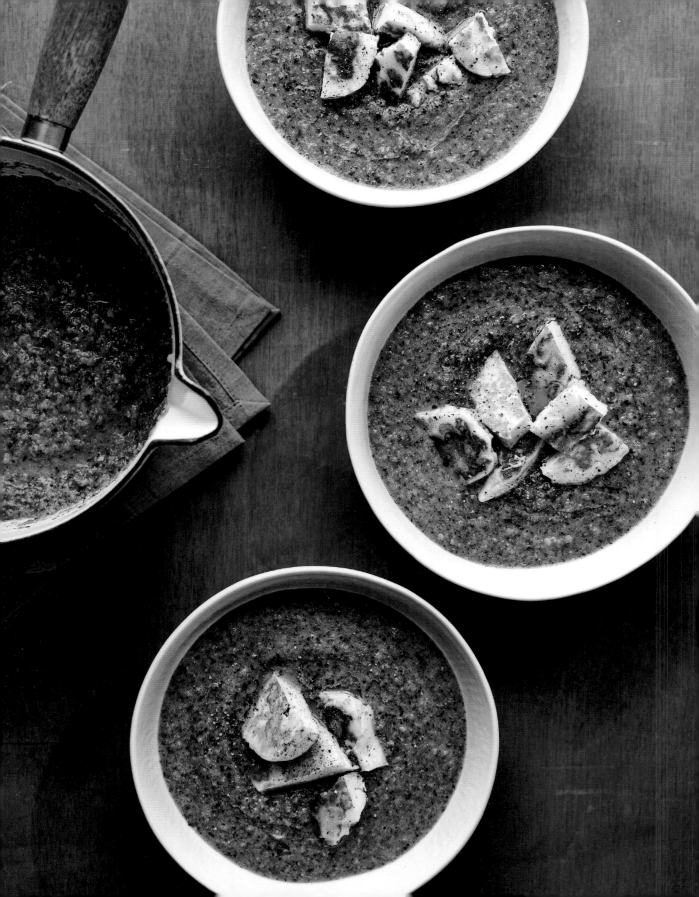

BROCCOLI SOUP WITH HALLOUMI CROUTONS

We all know broccoli is good for us, but it can taste a bit boring, can't it? Well, not when you blend it with lentils and spices in this gorgeous soup and top it with soft halloumi croutons. Squeaky little cheese, I love you!

SERVES 4–6

2 tbsp olive oil

2 onions, diced

6 garlic cloves, crushed

80g split red lentils, rinsed

1 litre vegetable stock (or chicken stock if not vegetarian)

6 sprigs of thyme, leaves picked

2 heads of broccoli (about 700g), cut into small florets

100g fresh or frozen spinach

juice of ½ lemon

225g halloumi cheese

salt and freshly ground black pepper

1 Heat 1 tablespoon of the oil in a medium saucepan over a medium heat. Once hot, add the onions and cook for about 10 minutes, stirring occasionally, until starting to brown.

2 Push the onions to one side, add the remaining oil to the pan and sprinkle in the crushed garlic. Cook until the garlic starts to turn golden, then stir it through the onions.

3 Add the rinsed lentils, stock and thyme leaves, bring to boil, then reduce to a simmer and cook for 15 minutes until the lentils are tender.

4 Add the broccoli and cook for a further 6–8 minutes until the broccoli is soft, then add the spinach and cover with a lid for a minute so the spinach can wilt/defrost. Stir in the lemon juice.

5 Use a stick blender to blitz about half of the soup, if you like it chunky, or go the whole way to get it really smooth. If you only have a free-standing blender, you can remove roughly half of the soup to your blender, blitz until smooth, then stir it back into the pan to get the chunky texture. You can loosen it with a bit of water to get it to your preferred consistency, if you like. Taste and season with salt and pepper, as needed.

6 Cut the halloumi into 5mm slices and fry in a dry frying pan over a high heat until golden underneath, then flip and cook on the other side until golden. Remove from the frying pan, let cool slightly, then cut into bite-sized chunks.

7 Divide the soup between bowls and garnish with the halloumi croutons.

JOE'S TIP

Split red lentils are super cheap to buy and cook really quickly – they are an easy way to make soups more filling and are excellent to have in the cupboard for a quick, protein- and fibre-packed lunch or supper.

BEEF CHILLI & TORTILLA SOUP

This is a very hearty soup – almost a stew. It's basically a classic spicy beef chilli in soup form! The home-made tortilla strips make a satisfying, crunchy garnish. I know you'll enjoy this one.

SERVES 4

1 tbsp light olive oil

1 onion, sliced

400g minced beef

200g roasted red peppers from a jar, rinsed and sliced into strips

400g tin of chopped tomatoes

400g tin of kidney beans, drained and rinsed

2 tsp chipotle paste (optional, but recommended) or 2 tsp smoked paprika

2 tsp dried oregano

1 tsp ground cumin

½ tsp cayenne pepper

1 beef stock cube

salt, to taste

Crispy Tortilla Strips

4 small tortillas, preferably corn, cut into 1cm-wide strips

1 tbsp light olive oil

To Serve

grated Cheddar cheese

fresh coriander leaves

natural yoghurt

hot sauce or thinly sliced green chillies

1 Preheat the oven to 200°C/180°C fan.

2 For the crispy tortilla strips, toss the tortilla strips with 1 tbsp oil on a baking tray. Bake for 4–6 minutes until slightly browned. They will crisp up as they cool.

3 Heat the oil in a large saucepan over a medium heat, add the onion and cook until golden, about 10 minutes. Add the beef and stir until no longer pink, scraping the bottom of the pan to incorporate any browned bits. Add the roasted pepper strips along with the tinned tomatoes, kidney beans, chipotle paste or smoked paprika, herbs and spices. Fill the tomato tin twice with water and add both to the pan, then crumble in the beef stock cube and stir together. Bring to the boil, then cover and reduce to a simmer. Cook for 30 minutes, stirring occasionally, so the flavours can develop. Taste and season with salt, if needed.

4 Divide the soup between 4 bowls and top with the tortilla strips, pushing them down slightly so some are submerged in the soup. Top with your choice of garnishes and serve.

FEEL GOOD FACT

Beef is rich in iron (key for healthy growth and development and for maintaining energy levels) and in vitamin B12 (for healthy function of the brain and nervous system).

HEARTY

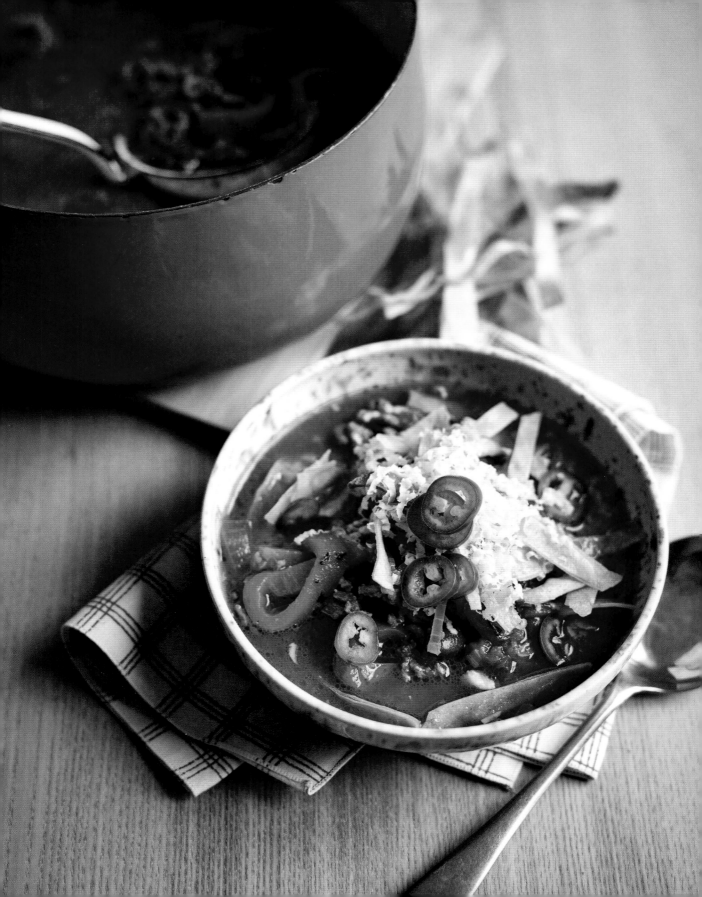

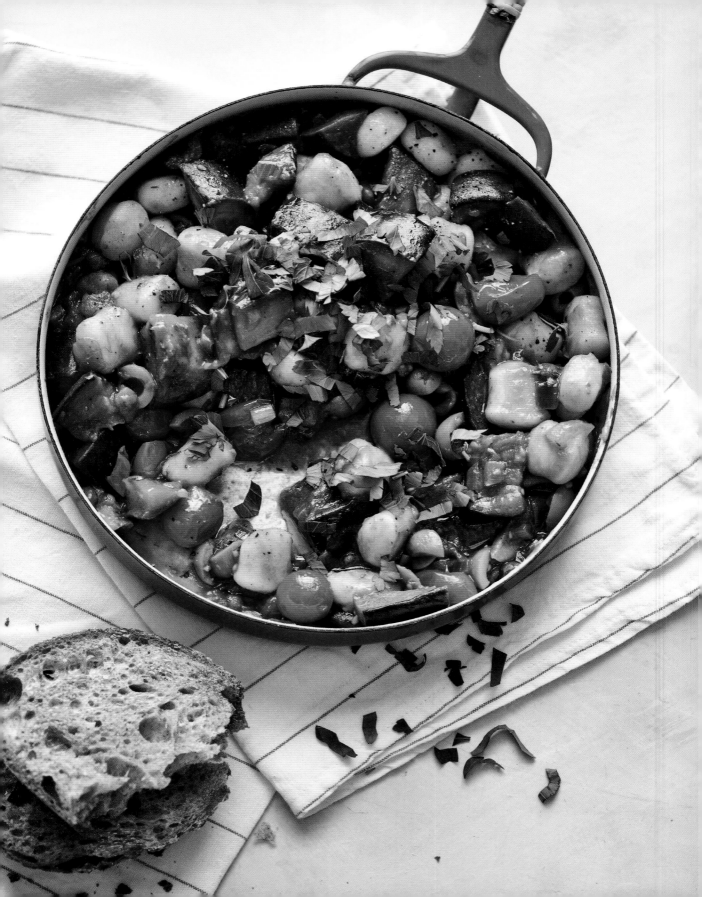

AUBERGINE, TOMATO & CAPER GNOCCHI

If you've not tried gnocchi before, this is your chance. I love them – they're a bit like a cross between a potato dumpling and pasta. They are easy to find now in most supermarkets, too. Here, they are coated in a tangy sauce of tomatoes, olives and capers, which is mixed with yummy aubergine.

SERVES 4

2 aubergines

2 tbsp light olive oil

1 red onion, diced

2 garlic cloves, crushed

400g tin of cherry tomatoes

1 tbsp capers

1 tbsp balsamic vinegar

1 tsp dried oregano

100g pitted green olives, roughly chopped

500g gnocchi

handful of flat-leaf parsley, roughly chopped

salt

1 Cut the aubergine into 3cm chunks and sprinkle with salt. Leave to sit on the chopping board for a few minutes to draw out some of the moisture from the aubergine (this makes it creamier when cooked), then dry on a clean tea towel.

2 Add the aubergine to a large, dry, non-stick frying pan over a medium heat and cook until it starts to brown. Add the olive oil and onion and cook until the onion has softened, around 5 minutes. Stir in the garlic and cook for 1 minute, then add the tomatoes, capers, balsamic vinegar, oregano and olives. Stir together and cook over a medium-low heat for 10 minutes until slightly thickened.

3 Meanwhile, bring a large pan of salted water to the boil. Add the gnocchi and cook according to the packet instructions.

4 Drain the gnocchi and tip into the pan of sauce, then stir for 1–2 minutes to help the sauce coat the pasta.

5 Divide between bowls and top with the chopped parsley.

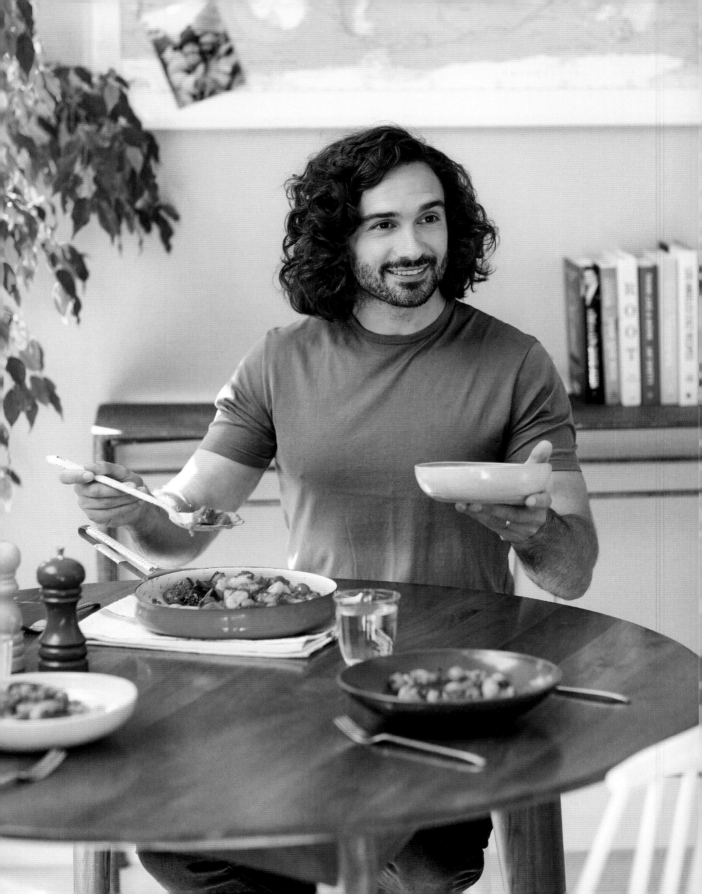

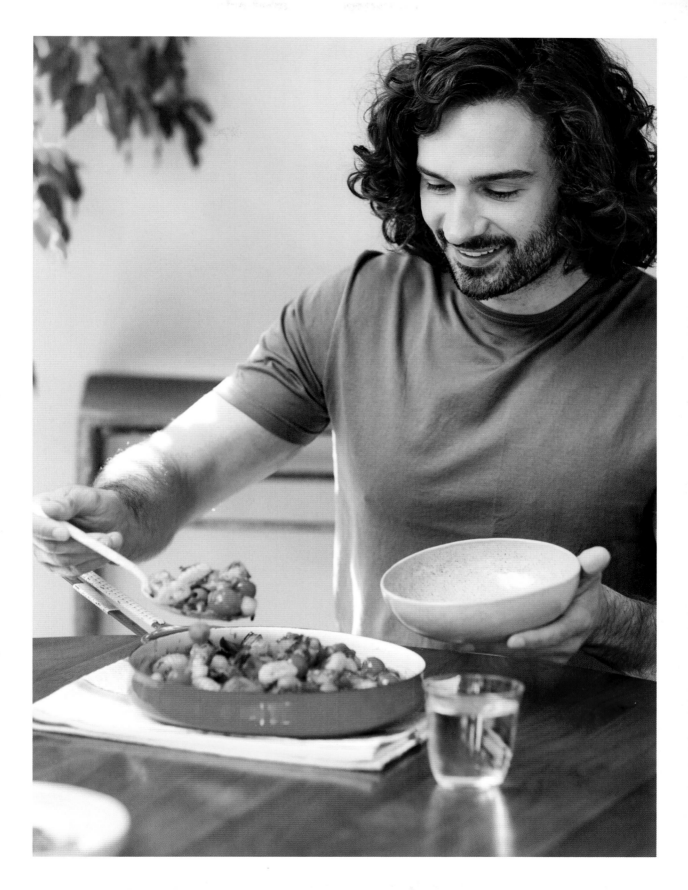

ROASTED TOFU, BEANS & MUSHROOMS WITH STICKY ORANGE SAUCE

Baking tofu gives it a really awesome, crispy outer layer. It's my favourite way to eat it and I love it with this sticky orange sauce made with dates. If you haven't eaten tofu before, I think this a great recipe for you to try.

SERVES 4

450g firm tofu

450g mixed mushrooms e.g. shiitake or chestnut

1 tbsp soy sauce

1 tsp sesame oil

1 tbsp cornflour

1 tsp Chinese five spice

1 tsp ground white pepper

2 tbsp panko breadcrumbs

pinch of salt

200g green beans, trimmed

2 tbsp light olive oil or melted, refined coconut oil

Sticky Orange Sauce

100g pitted dates

75ml soy sauce

2 garlic cloves, crushed

120ml orange juice (not from concentrate)

1 tsp cornflour

1 tsp apple cider vinegar

To Serve

400g cooked brown basmati rice

4 spring onions, thinly sliced

2 tbsp sesame seeds

1 Preheat the oven to 200°C/180°C fan.

2 Press the tofu by wrapping it in a clean tea towel and placing onto a chopping board. Place another board on top and weigh it down with a couple of cookbooks. Leave for 15–30 minutes to drain, then unwrap.

3 Cut any larger mushrooms in half or into quarters, then toss with the soy sauce and sesame oil on a rimmed baking tray. Roast for 30–40 minutes until they are shrunken and slightly crispy.

4 Cut the tofu into roughly 2cm cubes. Toss the cornflour, five spice, white pepper, breadcrumbs and salt in a bowl, then add the tofu and toss until coated. Tip onto a second baking tray along with the green beans, toss with the olive or coconut oil and bake for 20–25 minutes until the tofu is crisp.

5 To make the sauce, soak the pitted dates in boiling water for 15 minutes, then drain them, leaving about 2 tablespoons of soaking liquid in the jug. Blitz with a hand blender until smooth, then scrape the date paste into a small saucepan. Add the remaining sauce ingredients and stir over a high heat until the mixture starts to bubble and thicken slightly. Remove from the heat and allow to cool for a few minutes.

6 Serve the crispy tofu and roasted mushrooms with cooked brown rice, drizzled with the sauce and garnished with the spring onions and sesame seeds.

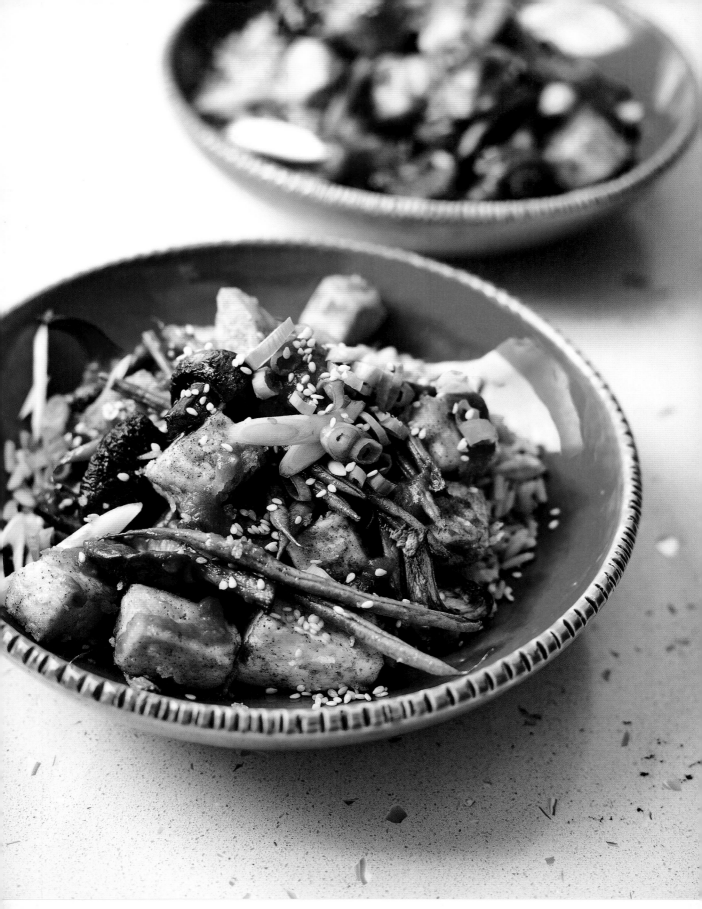

GARLIC CHICKEN & MUSHROOM TRAYBAKE

I love a traybake – everything cooks together in the same pan, which means less washing up, and that's always a win in my eyes. Cooking the chicken in with the rice means the rice gets flavoured with the meaty juices and the garlic-and-herb rub. The rice cooks perfectly and it's just gorgeous.

SERVES 4

300g mini portobello mushrooms, sliced

1 tbsp light olive oil

30g butter, softened

3 garlic cloves, crushed

handful of flat-leaf parsley,
   roughly chopped

3 sprigs of thyme, leaves picked

4 bone-in, skin-on chicken thighs

4 bone-in, skin-on chicken drumsticks

250g white basmati rice

1 chicken or vegetable stock cube

600ml boiling water

250g Tenderstem broccoli

salt

1 Preheat the oven to 200°C/180°C fan.

2 Toss the mushrooms with the olive oil and a pinch of salt in a deep, 23 x 33cm (or a similar size) roasting pan. Roast for 20 minutes until browned.

3 Meanwhile, mix the softened butter, garlic, parsley and thyme with a pinch of salt in a small bowl. Rub this mixture over the chicken thighs and drumsticks, then set aside.

4 Once the mushrooms are done, add the rice to the roasting pan, crumble over the stock cube and pour in the boiling water. Stir together to combine, then top with the chicken pieces. Cover the pan tightly with foil and bake for 30 minutes.

5 Remove the pan from the oven, remove the foil and scatter over the broccoli. Return to the oven, uncovered, for 15–20 minutes until the broccoli is tender and the chicken has browned.

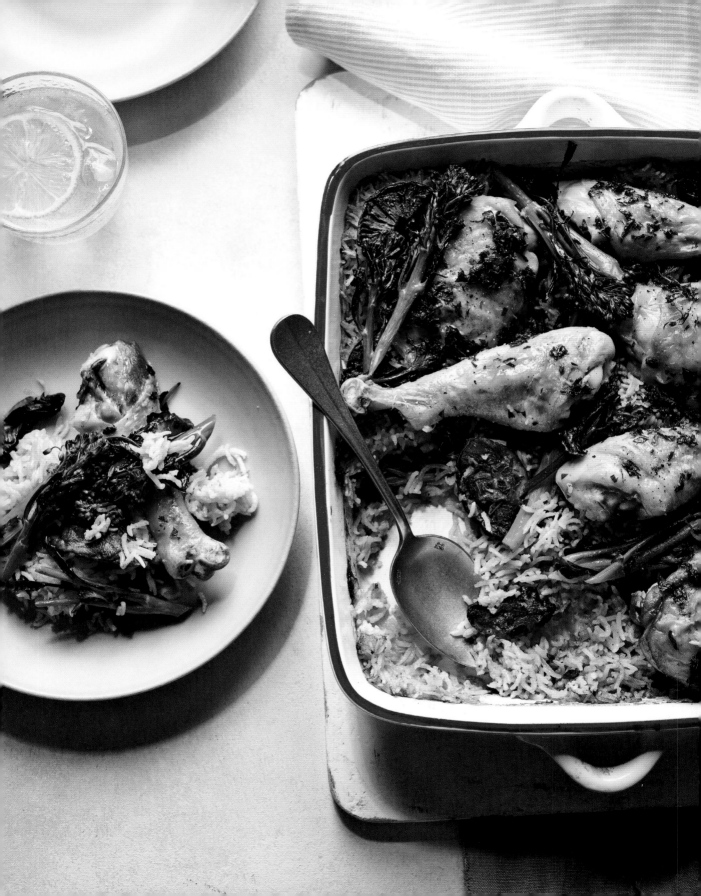

CHICKEN & SQUASH CURRY RAMEN

This is a really rich and comforting noodle dish – gently spiced and creamy from the coconut milk and butternut squash. It tastes absolutely wonderful. Defo give this one a go! Feel free to leave out the eggs, if they're not your thing.

SERVES 4

1½ tbsp coconut oil

1 butternut squash, peeled, seeds removed, cut into 2cm chunks

2 chicken thighs (around 300g) (or chicken breasts, if you prefer)

750ml chicken or vegetable stock

4 tbsp korma curry paste

2 tsp grated ginger

1 tsp ground cumin

1 tsp garam masala

400ml coconut milk

2 pak choi, trimmed, leaves separated

4 large eggs

250g medium egg noodles

2 spring onions, thinly sliced

soy sauce, to serve

JOE'S TIPS

- You can use other curry pastes for a different flavour or heat level. If you can get a quality laksa paste, or green or red Thai curry pastes, they all work really well, although you'll probably only need 2–3 tbsp as they tend to be stronger.
- To make this veggie, skip the chicken thighs and use veg stock. You can add some shiitake mushrooms to the broth along with the pak choi for extra texture.

1 In a large frying pan, melt the coconut oil over a medium-low heat. Add the squash and cover with a lid. Cook for 15 minutes, removing the lid every 3–5 minutes to stir. It should be browned all over and slightly soft.

2 Push the squash to the edges of the pan and add the chicken thighs. Cook until starting to brown underneath, then flip and cook on the other side until golden. Pour in the stock, bring to the boil, then reduce to a simmer. Cover the pan and cook for 15 minutes until the chicken is cooked through.

3 Remove the chicken thighs to a chopping board and shred with two forks. Set aside.

4 In a small frying pan, fry the curry paste with the ginger, cumin and garam masala over a medium heat, stirring until the paste thickens slightly. Pour this into the large frying pan and stir in along with the coconut milk. Add the pak choi, cover and cook for 3–4 minutes.

5 Bring a medium pan of water to the boil. Once boiling, reduce to a simmer and gently lower in the eggs. Cook for 5½ minutes. Remove with a slotted spoon to a bowl of cold water, then peel the eggs and set aside.

6 Keep the pan of water boiling and add the noodles, cooking according to the packet instructions.

7 Drain the noodles and divide between 4 noodle bowls. Ladle on the creamy broth and veg from the frying pan. Cut the eggs in half and top each bowl with a halved egg, some shredded chicken and sliced spring onions. Serve with soy sauce at the table for adjusting the salt level.

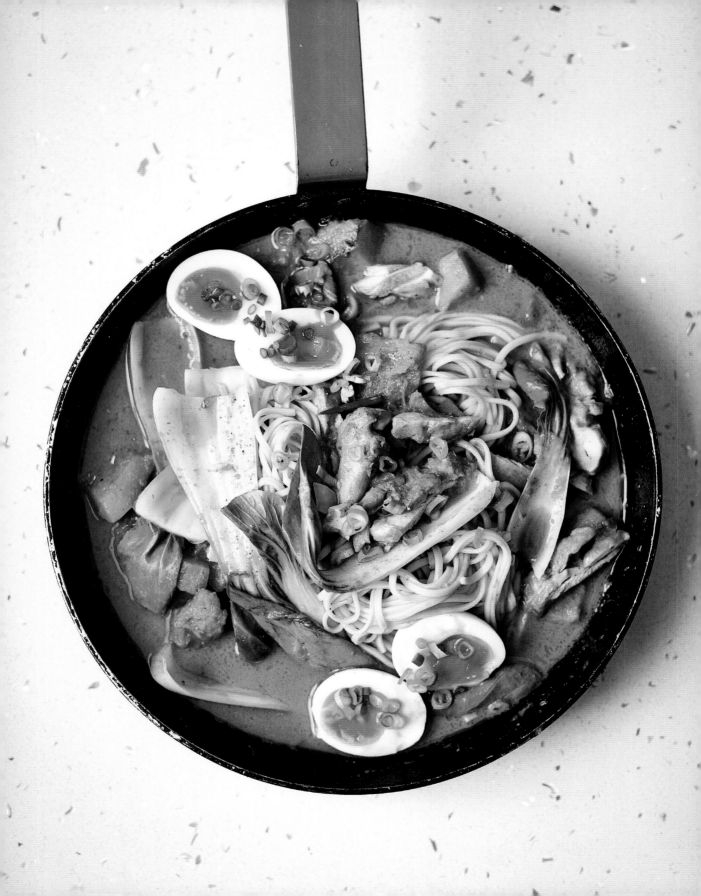

VEG-PACKED BOLOGNESE

You may be thinking, where's the minced beef in this recipe? Trust me, though, this method using a food processor means you won't miss the meat at all. The veggies all get blitzed up to a similar texture to mince and all the flavour of a classic rich Bolognese is still here. If you're not veggie, adding a beef stock cube means the sauce will have lots of meaty flavour; if you are veggie, use a vegetable stock cube and a bit of Marmite to get that savoury taste.

SERVES 6-8

3 tbsp olive oil

2 medium onions, roughly chopped

3 celery sticks, roughly chopped

3 medium carrots, roughly chopped

300g chestnut mushrooms

100g tomato purée concentrate (tomato paste)

400g tin of chopped tomatoes

250g pouch of cooked Puy lentils or 400g tin of cooked green lentils, drained

1 low-salt vegetable stock cube plus 1 tbsp Marmite (or 1 beef stock cube)

1 sprig rosemary

2 bay leaves

1 tsp dried oregano

1 tbsp balsamic vinegar

400g wholemeal spaghetti

salt

grated vegetarian hard cheese or Parmesan, to serve

JOE'S TIP

This is obviously a great recipe for batch cooking. Any leftovers can be kept in the fridge for up to 3 days or frozen for up to 3 months. You can use the leftovers to make a quick lasagne or even a shepherd's pie.

1 Heat the olive oil in a large saucepan over a low heat.

2 Add the onions to a food processor and pulse until finely chopped – don't take them too far or they'll become a purée! Scrape into the pan and stir to coat with the oil. Blitz the celery and carrots in the same way and add to the pan with the onions. You may need to blitz in batches.

3 Cook the veg over a medium heat with a pinch of salt, stirring often, until softened and translucent, around 5–7 minutes. Remove the veg from the pan to a large bowl and set aside.

4 Add the mushrooms to the food processor and pulse until finely chopped. Tip the mushrooms into the pan with another pinch of salt and cook on a medium-low heat. Stir often and cook until the mushrooms release their liquid and then dry out, around 10 minutes.

5 Add the cooked veg back to the pan along with the tomato purée, chopped tomatoes, lentils, stock cube, Marmite (if using), herbs and vinegar. Fill the tomato tin twice with water and add that to the pan, too. Stir together and let the mixture come to the boil. Once boiling, reduce the heat to low and cook for 1 hour, stirring every now and then to prevent it catching.

6 Meanwhile, cook your spaghetti in a large pan of salted, boiling water according to the packet instructions. Drain, reserving a small mugful of the pasta cooking water.

7 Remove and discard the rosemary sprig and bay leaves from the sauce. Mix a few large spoonfuls of the sauce into the cooked pasta, loosening with splashes of pasta water as needed.

8 Divide the pasta between 4 bowls and top with more sauce and a grating of cheese.

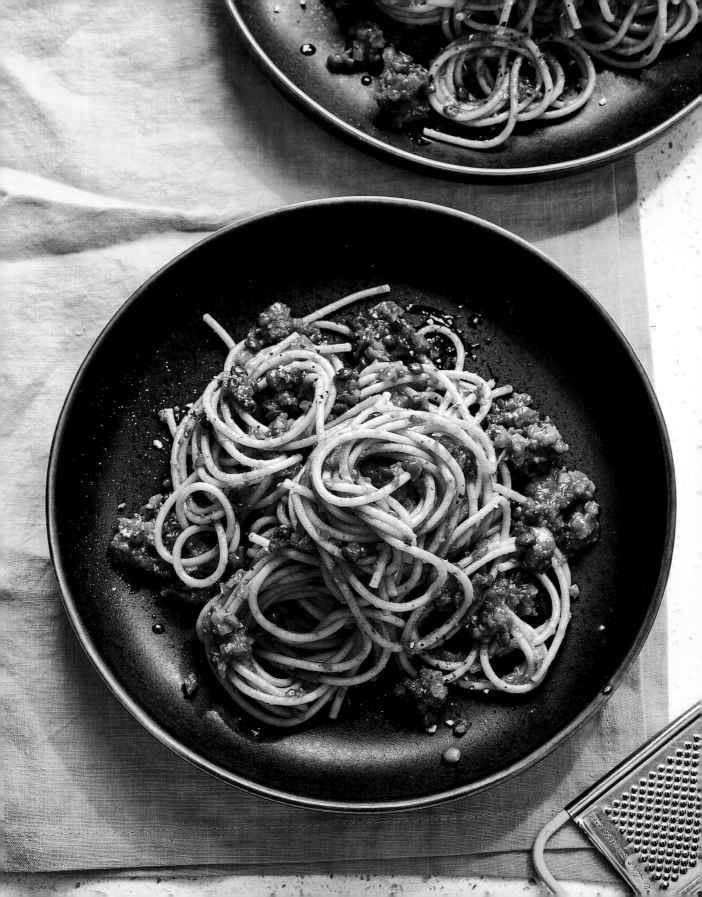

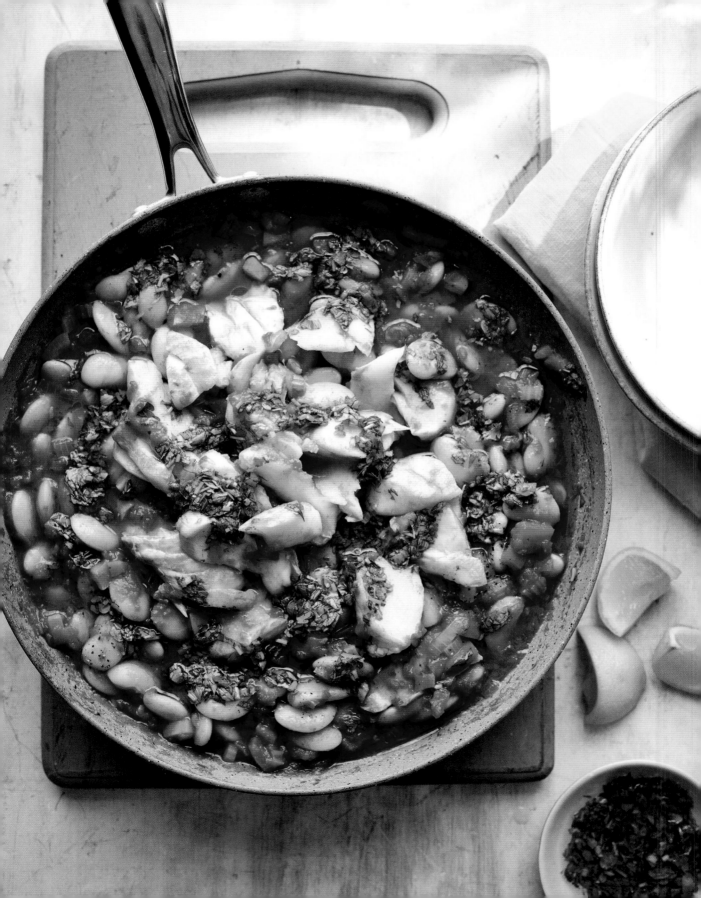

SMOKY COD, TOMATO & PEPPER STEW

This is a super-hearty stew that's packed full of goodness and has so much flavour. If you're looking for something to fill you and your family up, this recipe is ideal. I like to serve it with a slice of crusty bread on the side to soak up all the spicy, juicy flavours of the sauce.

SERVES 4

2 tbsp light olive oil

2 onions, diced

2 medium carrots, diced

2 celery sticks, diced

2 red or orange bell peppers, seeds removed, diced

pinch of salt

2 x 400g tins of chopped tomatoes

¼–½ tsp chilli flakes

2 tsp smoked paprika

2 tbsp soy sauce

1 vegetable or chicken stock cube

2 x 400g tins of butter beans

280g skinless cod fillets or other white fish

lemon wedges, to serve

Parsley Pesto

30g fresh flat-leaf parsley

2 tbsp extra-virgin olive oil

1 tbsp lemon juice

1 garlic clove, crushed

pinch of salt

1 Heat the oil in a heavy-based saucepan over a medium-low heat, add the onions, carrots, celery and peppers with the salt, and cook for 15 minutes until the vegetables have softened.

2 Add the chopped tomatoes, chilli flakes, smoked paprika and soy sauce, then crumble in the stock cube. Add the tins of butter beans along with their liquid and stir together. Bring to the boil, then reduce the heat to low and cook for 1 hour, stirring occasionally.

3 Add the cod to the pan, cover with a lid and cook for 5–10 minutes until the cod flakes apart easily. Remove the cod from the pot and flake it apart, then stir back into the stew.

4 To make the parsley pesto, chop the parsley as finely as possible and add to a bowl with the remaining pesto ingredients. Stir to combine. Alternatively, pulse the pesto ingredients together in a small food processor.

5 Serve the stew topped with the pesto, with lemon wedges on the side for squeezing over.

PEANUT BUTTER & COCONUT VEGETABLE CURRY

Calling all peanut butter lovers. This curry is the one. Loads of veg all thrown into a beautiful coconut and peanut curry sauce. It tastes incredible just as it is, but you can also serve it with some jasmine or basmati rice, if you like.

SERVES 4

1 tbsp coconut oil

2 onions, diced

6 garlic cloves, crushed

1 tbsp grated fresh ginger

2 red chillies, seeds removed, finely chopped

2 tsp cumin seeds

2 tsp coriander seeds

600ml water

400g tin of light coconut milk

4 tbsp smooth peanut butter

1 tsp ground turmeric

2 tsp runny honey or maple syrup

1 vegetable stock cube

400g new potatoes, halved

400g cauliflower, cut into small florets

2 x 400g tins of chickpeas, drained and rinsed

2 tsp garam masala

salt, to taste

To Serve

500g cooked brown basmati rice

1 lime, cut into wedges

1 Heat the oil in a large saucepan over a medium heat, add the onions and cook for 7–10 minutes until softened. Stir in the garlic, ginger, chillies, cumin and coriander seeds, and cook for 1 minute, then add the water, coconut milk, peanut butter, turmeric and honey or maple syrup, and crumble in the vegetable stock cube. Bring to a simmer, then add the potatoes, cauliflower and chickpeas. Bring back to a simmer, cover and cook for 15–20 minutes until the vegetables have softened.

2 Uncover and stir in the garam masala to finish. Season to taste.

3 Serve the curry with the cooked rice, with lime wedges for squeezing over.

FEEL GOOD FACT

Peanut butter is cheap and nutrient dense – it provides healthy fats, protein and fibre, which help control blood sugar levels and keep you feeling fuller for longer.

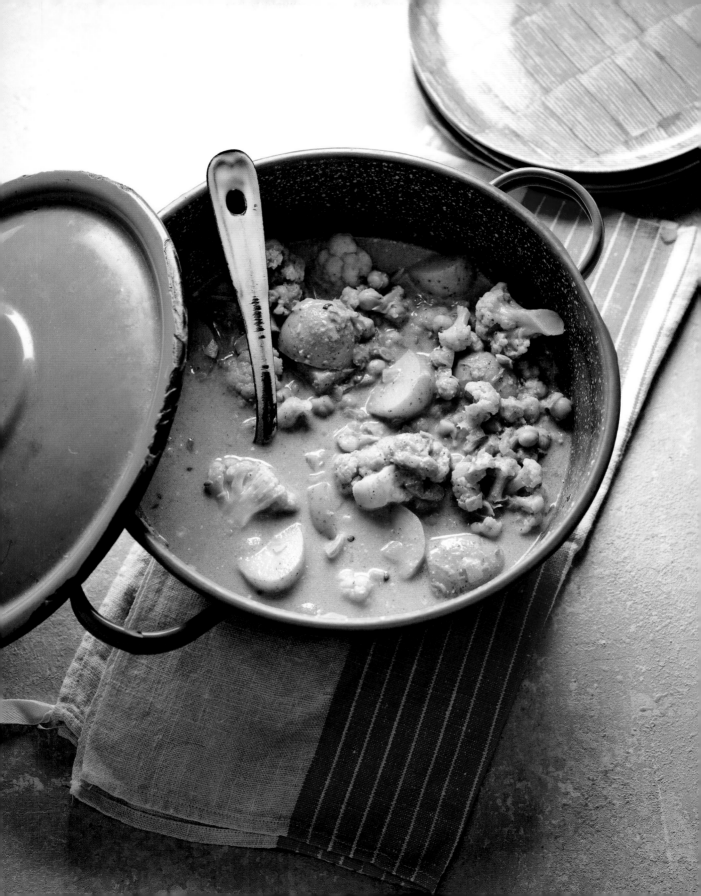

RED LENTIL DAL & QUICK APPLE PICKLE

A great dish for those days when you want to avoid meat and try something veggie. Red lentils are a great plant-based source of protein, gentle on your gut and super cheap, so it's always a good idea to have some handy in the cupboard. This makes a really creamy curry that's great scooped up with some wholemeal flatbreads or pitas. Yummy!

SERVES 4

2 tbsp coconut oil

1 red onion, diced

2 tsp grated fresh ginger

3 medium carrots, finely diced

200g split red lentils, rinsed

750ml water

400g tin of chopped tomatoes

½ tsp ground turmeric

½–1 tsp chilli flakes

2 tsp cumin seeds

2 tsp black mustard seeds

4 garlic cloves, thinly sliced

2 tsp garam masala

salt, to taste

Quick Apple Pickle

1 apple

2 tbsp apple cider vinegar

2 spring onions, thinly sliced

handful of coriander leaves, finely chopped

pinch of salt

To Serve

handful of coriander leaves, roughly chopped

natural yoghurt (if not vegan)

wholemeal flatbreads or pita breads, warmed

cooked rice (optional)

1 Heat 1 tablespoon of the coconut oil in a large saucepan over a medium heat until melted. Add the diced onion and cook for about 10 minutes, stirring occasionally, until it is starting to brown. Stir in the grated ginger, and cook for 1–2 minutes to remove the raw taste. Add the carrots, lentils, water, tomatoes, turmeric and chilli flakes, bring to the boil, then reduce the heat and leave to simmer for 25–30 minutes until the lentils are tender.

2 Meanwhile, make the quick apple pickle. Core the apple and dice it into small chunks. Toss into a bowl with the vinegar, spring onions, coriander and salt, stir together to combine and set aside.

3 Once the lentils are cooked, heat the remaining tablespoon of coconut oil in a small frying pan over a medium heat. Add the cumin seeds, mustard seeds and sliced garlic, and cook until the garlic starts to become slightly golden. Remove from the heat and pour the contents of the pan into the pot of lentils along with the garam masala. Stir together, taste, and season with salt as needed.

4 Serve the lentils with a sprinkling of roughly chopped coriander, the apple pickle, a dollop of yoghurt, if using, and some flatbreads. You can also serve it with rice, if you like.

HEARTY

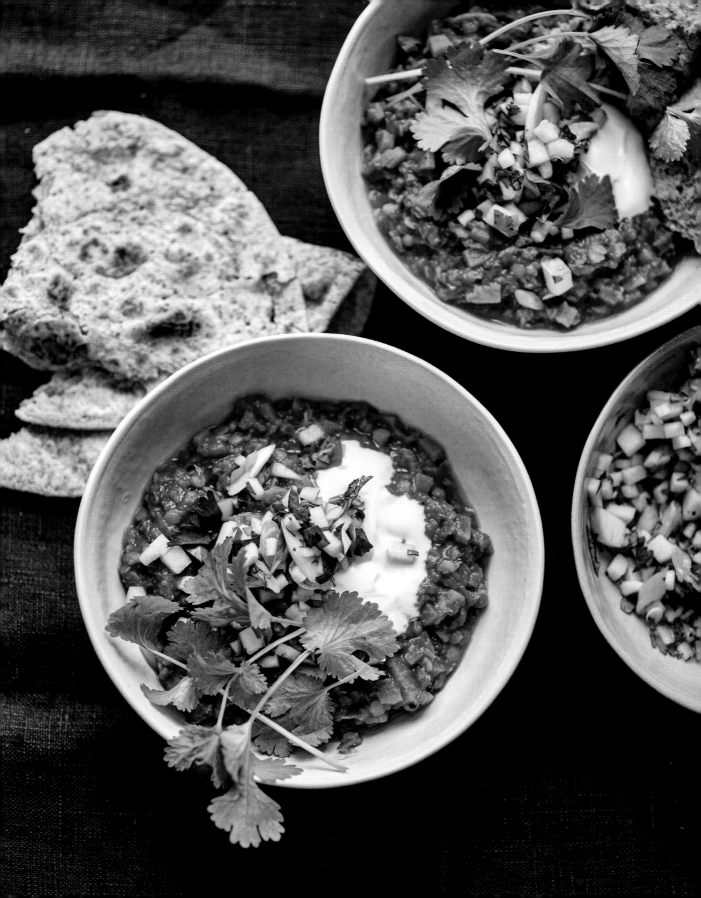

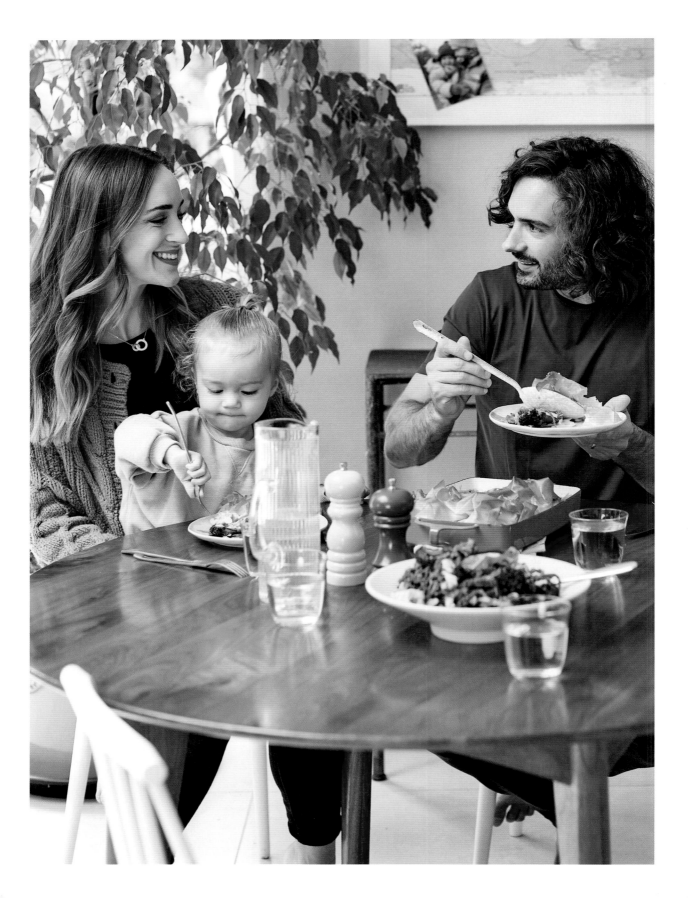

7

CROWD-
PLEASERS

food to wow family and friends

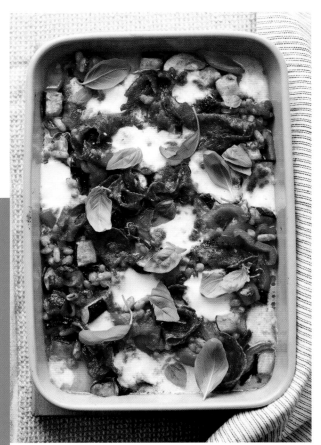

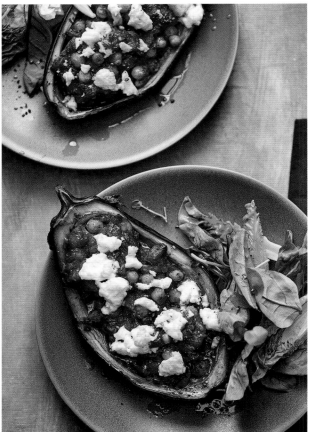

Eating with my loved ones is one of my all-time feel good activities. Who doesn't love a get-together?! I think there's nothing better than getting a group of mates or family together to eat great food. And, of course, I want everyone to be wowed by what's on the table.

These are meals that will feed a family with leftovers or a large group of friends with ease. They all have a bit of wow factor, too, so that when you put that dish in the middle of the table, your mates can't fail to be impressed. Some of the recipes are for larger groups of up to 6 or 8, but can easily be halved, if needed. Alternatively, leftovers can be refrigerated or popped in the freezer for another time. Other recipes will feed 4 generously and can be doubled or tripled to feed larger crowds.

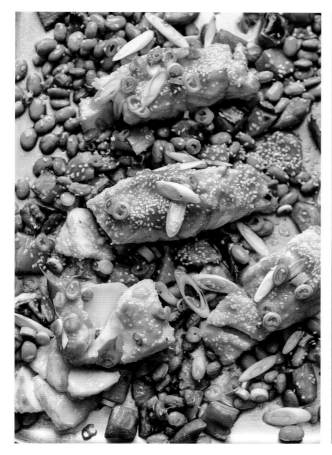

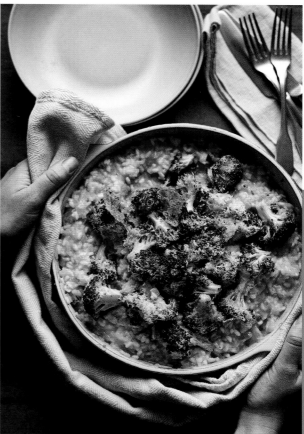

To keep things simple, I love a batch-cook. If you've got mates over for the weekend, cooking up a big pot of something that will give you leftovers for a family lunch or dinner the next day or later in the week is a win-win for me! Try out my awesome chilli recipes on pages 238 and 240 – they're just the ticket. One for the meat-eaters and an equally amazing one for the veggies.

Or, if you're after something a bit more elegant for a special occasion, you've got to check out the Moussaka-style Stuffed Aubergines on page 243. They're delicious and definitely have a bit of the X-factor. The Baked Paella-style Rice on page 244 is another favourite of mine for something special, and the filo-topped Chicken, Cauli, Leek and Bean Pie on page 262 just HAS to be tried. I think it's AMAZING and I know you will too!

SLOW-COOKED BEEF & BUTTERNUT SQUASH CHILLI

I love things that are easy to batch cook, because it covers you for lunch or dinner the following day. It really does set you up for a healthy week, so it's something I like to do on weekends. This slow-cooked beef chilli is absolutely delicious and tastes great served with rice or even on top of some pasta.

SERVES 8

2 tbsp light olive oil

2 red onions, sliced about 3mm thick

2 medium carrots, diced

3 celery sticks, diced

750g beef (silverside, brisket or other slow-cooking joints)

2 x 400g tins of black beans

400g tin of chopped tomatoes

250ml beef stock

3 tbsp soy sauce

2 tsp ground cumin

2 tsp smoked paprika

2 tsp dried oregano

1 tsp ground cinnamon

¼ tsp ground cloves

1 tsp sugar

1 medium butternut squash, peeled, seeds removed, diced into 3cm chunks (or 3 medium sweet potatoes, peeled and chopped)

To Serve

cooked brown rice

natural yoghurt

fresh coriander, roughly chopped

lime wedges

hot sauce

1 Preheat the oven to 170°C/150°C fan.

2 Set an ovenproof casserole dish over a medium heat and add the olive oil. Once hot, add the onions, carrots and celery, and cook for about 10 minutes, stirring often, until the vegetables have softened. Remove the vegetables to a plate and set aside.

3 Add the beef to the dish and brown on all sides, then return the vegetables along with the black beans and the liquid from the tins, the tomatoes, beef stock, soy sauce, spices and sugar. Stir together and cover with a lid, then transfer to the oven and roast for 3 hours.

4 Remove the dish from the oven and add the diced butternut squash. If it's looking too dry, pour in 250ml water. Return to the oven, covered, and roast for a further 2–3 hours. It's ready when the meat easily falls apart when poked with a fork. Check on the beef about 30 minutes before it's done – if it looks as though there's too much liquid, remove the lid for the rest of the cooking time.

5 Remove the dish from the oven and shred the beef using two forks. Stir the shredded beef into the sauce.

6 Serve the chilli hot with rice, a bit of yoghurt and some coriander. You can splash on some lime juice and hot sauce too, if you like.

JOE'S TIP

This makes a double batch and is freezer friendly! Eat the leftovers for lunch or cool, pop into a freezer-safe container, and freeze for up to 3 months. Use the chilli as a base for enchiladas, nachos or as a filling for tacos.

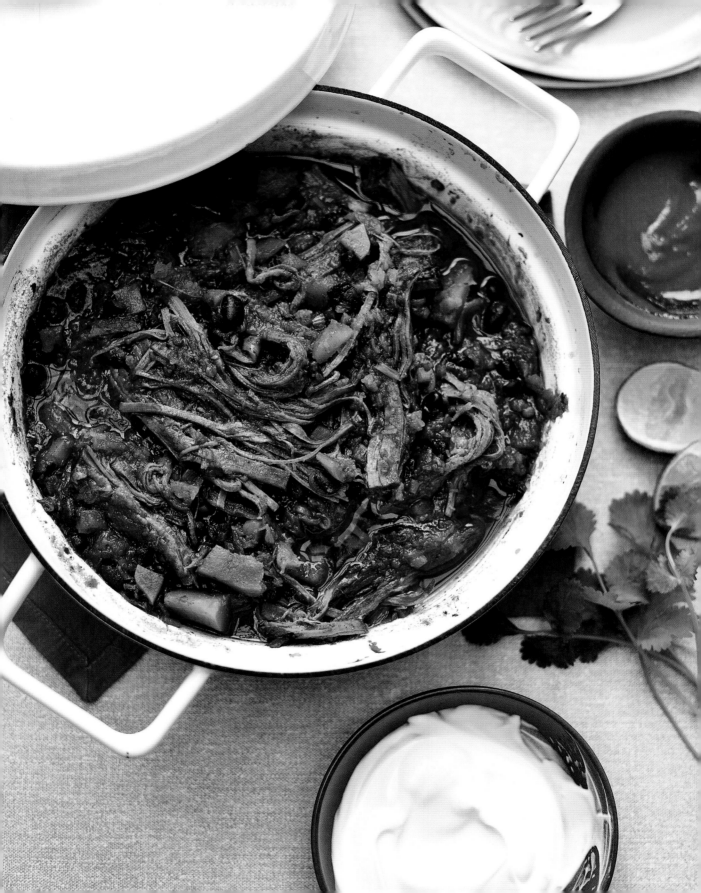

THE BEST VEGGIE CHILLI

This is the ultimate chilli – packed full of different veg and two types of bean. The Marmite and soy sauce give it that savoury, meaty flavour, but it's 100% vegan. It's so easy and cheap to make and, best of all, you can batch cook it and store it in the freezer – perfect to whip out at those times when you can't be bothered to cook.

SERVES 4–6

2 tbsp light olive oil

2 onions, diced

2 carrots, diced

400g tin of black beans

400g tin of kidney beans

400g tin of chopped tomatoes

200g frozen sliced peppers

2 tsp dried oregano

2 tsp ground cumin

2 tsp ground coriander

1 tsp ground cinnamon

1 tsp smoked paprika

½ tsp cayenne pepper

1 tbsp Marmite or soy sauce

1 tbsp apple cider vinegar

1 tsp sugar

400g tin of lentils, drained and rinsed

salt, to taste

To Serve

500g cooked brown rice

natural yoghurt (or plant-based yoghurt if vegan)

fresh coriander, roughly chopped

lime wedges

1 Heat the oil in a large saucepan over a medium heat, add the onions and carrots with a pinch of salt, then cook for around 10 minutes, stirring occasionally, until softened. Add both tins of beans along with the liquid from the tins to the pan, then tip in the chopped tomatoes, frozen peppers, herbs and spices, Marmite/soy sauce, apple cider vinegar and sugar. Fill the tomato tin with water and add that to the pan, too. Bring to the boil over a high heat, then reduce the heat to low and cook for 1 hour, stirring every 15 minutes or so to prevent it sticking and burning.

2 Stir in the drained lentils and continue to cook on low for a final 15–30 minutes. Taste and season with salt, if needed.

3 Serve the chilli with rice and top with yoghurt, coriander and a squeeze of lime, as you like.

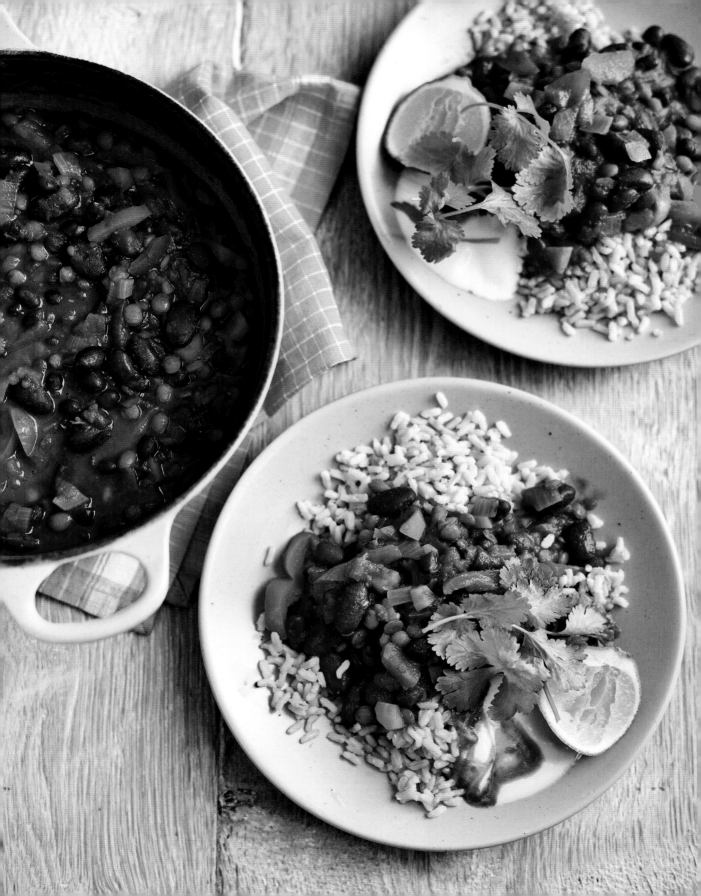

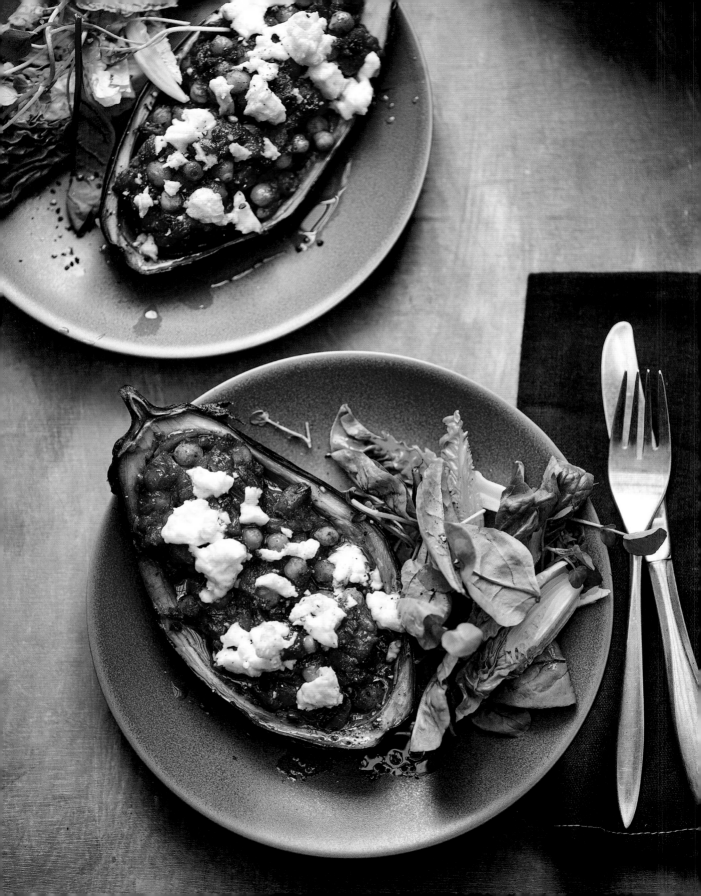

MOUSSAKA-STYLE STUFFED AUBERGINES

It's a super-yummy taste sensation going on right here. I've filled delicious aubergines with a Greek-style stuffing influenced by the flavours of moussaka. With plenty of nutritious chickpeas and tomatoes in the tasty lamb stuffing and topped with some creamy baked feta, it's a great dish for serving to friends when you want to impress!

SERVES 4

4 medium aubergines (get the chunkiest ones you can)

2 tbsp light olive oil, plus extra for brushing

1 red onion, diced

250g minced lamb

400g tin of chickpeas, drained and rinsed

400g tin of chopped tomatoes

1 tbsp red wine vinegar

3 sprigs of fresh thyme, leaves picked

2 tsp ground cinnamon

2 tsp dried oregano

200g feta cheese

salt

VARIATIONS

- You can use veggie mince in this recipe instead of the lamb. Just add 1 extra tablespoon of olive oil along with the veggie mince when frying it off.
- For a flavour boost, stir a heaped tablespoon of harissa paste into the mince mixture just before you scoop it into the aubergine halves.

1 Preheat the oven to 200°C/180°C fan.

2 Cut the aubergines in half down their lengths, then use a spoon to scoop the inner flesh from each half, leaving a border about 1cm thick (keep the flesh to one side). Brush the insides of the hollowed-out aubergines with a bit of olive oil, then place on a baking tray and bake for 20 minutes until softened.

3 Meanwhile, roughly chop the flesh scooped from the centre of the aubergines and sprinkle with a bit of salt. Set aside for 5 minutes to release some water.

4 Heat a non-stick frying pan over a medium heat and add the chopped aubergine flesh to the dry pan. Cook until it starts to brown in some places, then add 1 tablespoon of the oil and cook for about 5 minutes until well browned. Tip out of the pan into a bowl and set aside.

5 Heat the remaining tablespoon of oil in the same pan, add the onion and cook for about 5 minutes until softened. Add the lamb mince, breaking it up in the pan and stirring occasionally until browned. Stir in the chickpeas, tomatoes, vinegar, thyme, cinnamon and oregano. Cook for 10 minutes, or until reduced and thick. Stir the cooked chopped aubergine back in. Taste and season with salt as needed.

6 Divide the mixture between the baked aubergine halves. Crumble the feta and sprinkle it over the aubergines, then return them to the oven for 40–45 minutes until the feta has slightly browned and the aubergine skins are very soft.

BAKED PAELLA-STYLE RICE

I think paella is one of the greatest creations ever – so much going on, so many flavours and textures. I first tried it in Barcelona when I was a teenager and fell in love with it. This is a really easy way of cooking it, too, and it comes out perfectly.

SERVES 4

1 tbsp light olive oil

2 onions, diced

75g chorizo, diced

250g frozen sliced peppers

4 boneless, skinless chicken thighs, diced

250g arborio rice

100g cherry tomatoes, quartered

400ml boiling water

3 garlic cloves, crushed

1 chicken stock cube

2 tsp smoked paprika

¼ tsp ground turmeric

150g frozen peas

225g frozen cooked jumbo prawns, defrosted

handful of flat-leaf parsley, roughly chopped

4 lemon wedges

1 Preheat the oven to 240°C/220°C fan.

2 Add the oil, onions and chorizo to a deep 23 x 33cm (or a similar size) roasting tin. Bake for 7–10 minutes until the golden fat has started oozing out from the chorizo.

3 Remove from the oven, stir in the peppers and chicken, then return to the oven for a further 10 minutes.

4 Turn the oven down to 200°C/180°C fan.

5 Remove from the oven, add the rice and cherry tomatoes to the tin and mix in. In a jug, combine the boiling water, garlic, stock cube, smoked paprika and turmeric. Stir together to dissolve the stock cube, then pour into the tin. Cover tightly with kitchen foil and bake for 30 minutes until the rice is cooked.

6 Remove from the oven, remove the foil and stir in the peas and prawns, then return to the oven, uncovered, for 5 minutes to warm through.

7 Remove from the oven and garnish with the parsley. Serve with lemon wedges for squeezing.

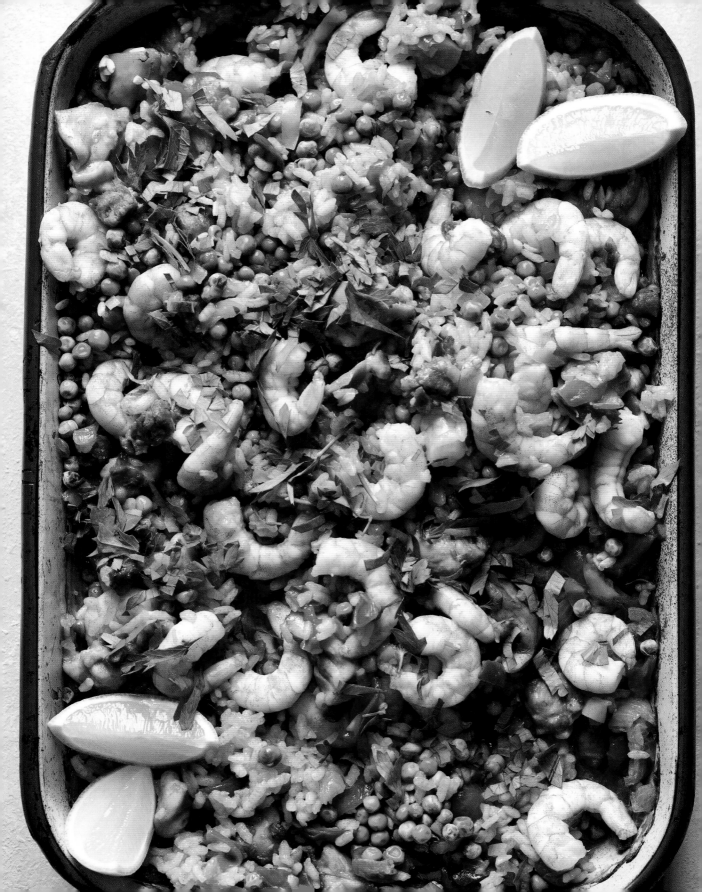

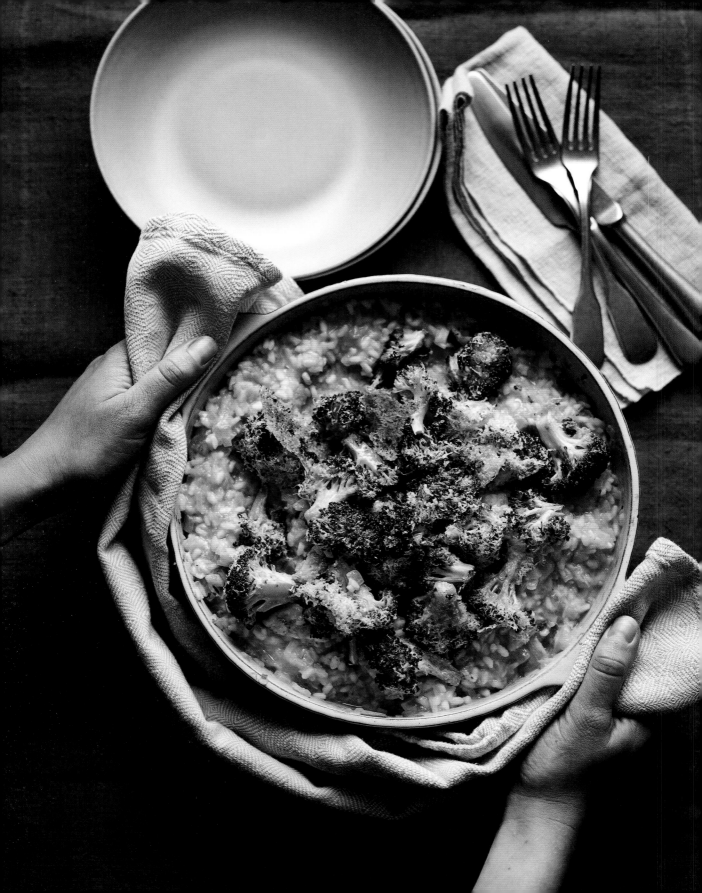

BAKED SQUASH RISOTTO WITH CRISPY CHEESY BROCCOLI

This recipe is an absolute joke – in the best way. It tastes unbelievable with the crispy cheesy broccoli on top. I promise, whoever is lucky enough to taste this one will be asking for seconds.

SERVES 4

1 small butternut squash, peeled, seeds removed, cut into 3cm chunks

3 tbsp light olive oil

1 small head of broccoli, cut into small florets

1 tsp garlic granules

20g vegetarian hard cheese or Parmesan, finely grated

1 large or 2 small onions, finely diced

3 celery sticks, finely diced

300g arborio rice

1 chicken or vegetable stock cube

900ml boiling water

4 sprigs of thyme, leaves picked

2 tbsp reduced-fat crème fraîche

1 tbsp lemon juice

salt

1 Preheat the oven to 200°C/180°C fan. Place one oven rack in the top third of the oven and a second rack on the lowest third. Line a large baking tray with baking paper.

2 Toss the butternut squash with 1 tablespoon of the oil on the baking tray and roast in the top third of the oven for 30 minutes until soft. Remove from the tray to a bowl and mash into a rough purée.

3 Add the broccoli to the tray and drizzle with 1 tablespoon of the oil. Sprinkle on the garlic granules and grated cheese and return to the top third of the oven for 15 minutes until crisp.

4 Meanwhile, place an ovenproof pan or casserole dish over a medium heat and add the remaining tablespoon of oil, the onion and celery. Cook over a medium-low heat for about 10 minutes, stirring occasionally, until softened. Add the rice and stir for a minute to toast slightly. Crumble in the stock cube, pour in the boiling water and add the thyme leaves. Stir together and bring to a simmer, then cover with a lid and transfer to the lower shelf of the oven to bake for 15–20 minutes until the rice is just cooked.

5 Remove from the oven and take off the lid. Stir in the butternut squash purée, crème fraîche and lemon juice. Taste and season with salt, as needed.

6 Divide between 4 bowls and top with the crispy broccoli.

TRAY-BAKED PORK FAJITAS

Fajitas are such a fun and messy way of eating together with family or friends. You get all the tasty ingredients together on the table and can have fun building your own perfect fajita. This recipe also works well with chicken or quick-cook beef strips.

SERVES 4

250g cherry tomatoes, halved

3 bell peppers, seeds removed, thinly sliced

3 red onions, quartered

1 tbsp light olive oil

pinch of salt

400g pork tenderloin, cut into short
  1cm strips

4 tsp fajita spice mix (see below)

40g tomato purée concentrate
  (tomato paste)

Fajita Spice Mix

2 tsp smoked paprika

2 tsp ground coriander

2 tsp ground cumin

1 tsp dried oregano

1 tsp chilli powder

1 tsp garlic granules

½ tsp granulated sugar

½ tsp salt

To Serve

8 wholemeal tortillas

½ head of iceberg lettuce, finely shredded

natural yoghurt

hot sauce

1 Preheat the oven to 200°C/180°C fan.

2 Mix together the fajita spice mix ingredients and set aside. This makes more than you need – the extra can be stored in an airtight jar for the next time you make this!

3 Toss the tomatoes, peppers and onions with the oil and a pinch of salt on a large baking tray. Roast for 30–40 minutes until the vegetables have started to caramelise.

4 Remove the tray from the oven. Mix the pork strips with the fajita spice mix and tomato purée, then scatter over the veg on the tray. Return to the oven for a further 20 minutes until the pork is cooked through.

5 Warm the tortillas according to the packet instructions.

6 Serve the pork and vegetables with the warm tortillas and have the lettuce, yoghurt and hot sauce in bowls on the table for everyone to help themselves.

JOE'S TIP

Making your own spice mix is not only cheaper, but also means you can control the amount of salt and sugar going into it. If you make a big batch and keep it in a jar, it'll cut down your prep time whenever you make fajitas.

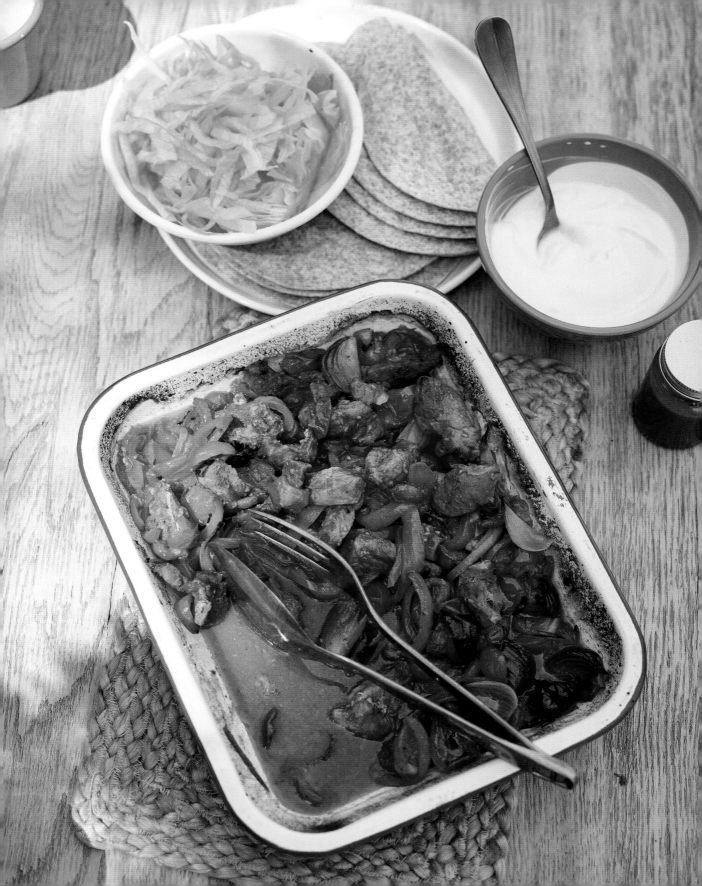

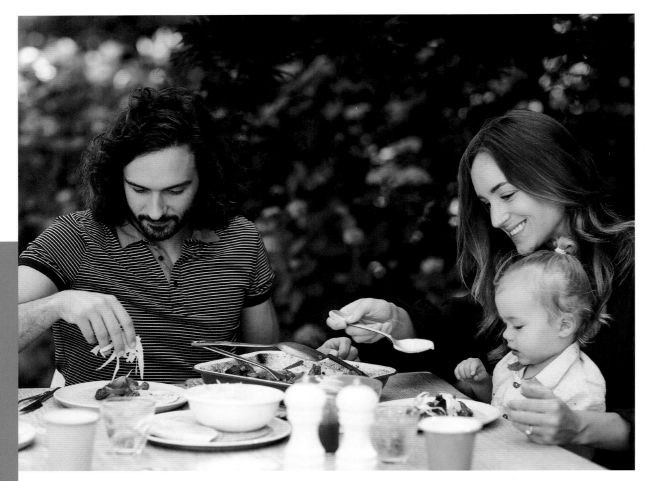

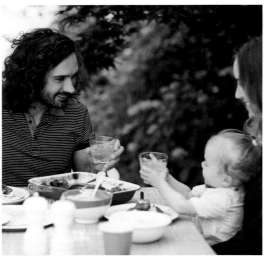

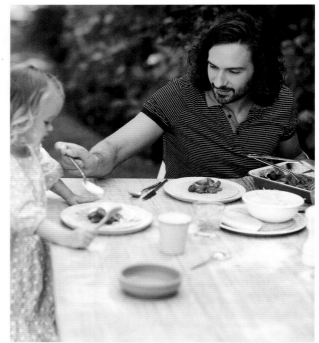

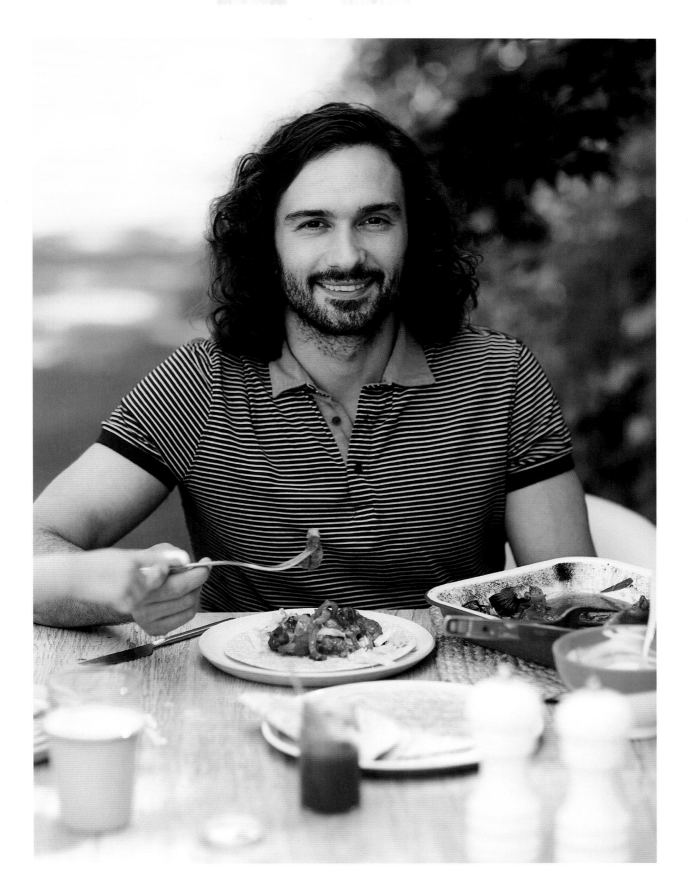

CHICKEN & CHICKPEA TAGINE WITH GREEN OLIVES, APRICOTS & LEMON

This is a really vibrant and tasty recipe. Once prepped and on the hob you can put your feet up and relax. Make sure you choose on-the-bone chicken thighs that still have the skin on – they provide a deep, rich flavour to the broth.

SERVES 4

2 tbsp olive oil

8 bone-in, skin-on chicken thighs

2 onions, peeled, sliced 3mm thick

3 garlic cloves, finely grated

2 red peppers, seeds removed, cut into wedges

250ml chicken stock

2 tsp ground cumin

1 tsp smoked paprika

½ tsp ground turmeric

½ tsp ground ginger

1 cinnamon stick

400g tin of chickpeas, drained and rinsed

160g pitted green olives

6 strips of pared lemon zest (use a vegetable peeler)

80g dried apricots, roughly chopped

To Serve

4 wholemeal flatbreads or 240g couscous

2 tbsp sesame seeds

30g fresh flat-leaf parsley, chopped

1 In a wide, deep pan or a casserole dish, heat 1 tablespoon of the oil over a medium heat. Add the chicken, skin-side down, and cook until golden underneath, then flip and cook the other side until golden. You may need to do this in batches if your pan isn't very wide. Remove the chicken to a plate and set aside.

2 Add the remaining olive oil to the pan with the onions and cook, stirring often, until they start to soften, around 5 minutes. Add the garlic and peppers and continue to cook for 5–7 minutes until the onions are beginning to brown. Add the chicken stock and scrape up any browned bits from the bottom of the pot. Stir in the spices, followed by the chickpeas, olives, lemon zest, apricots and cooked chicken. Bring to the boil, then reduce the heat to low and cover the pot with a lid. Leave to simmer for 30–40 minutes until the chicken is tender and cooked through.

3 Meanwhile, if serving with couscous, prepare according to the packet instructions and set aside. If serving with flatbreads, warm them up.

4 Place the sesame seeds in a small, dry frying pan and toast over a medium-high heat until golden and fragrant. Remove to a bowl quickly so they don't burn and set aside.

5 Top the cooked tagine with the toasted sesame seeds and chopped parsley, then serve with the warmed flatbreads or cooked couscous.

FEEL GOOD FACT

Olives are high in vitamin E, which helps maintain healthy skin and supports the immune system, and they also contain healthy fats, which may support heart health.

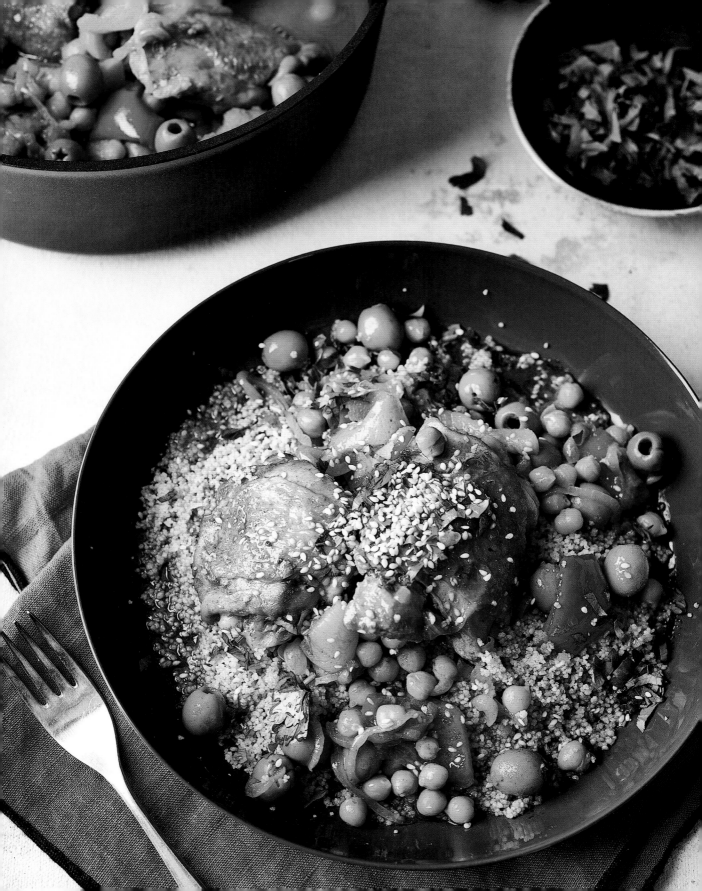

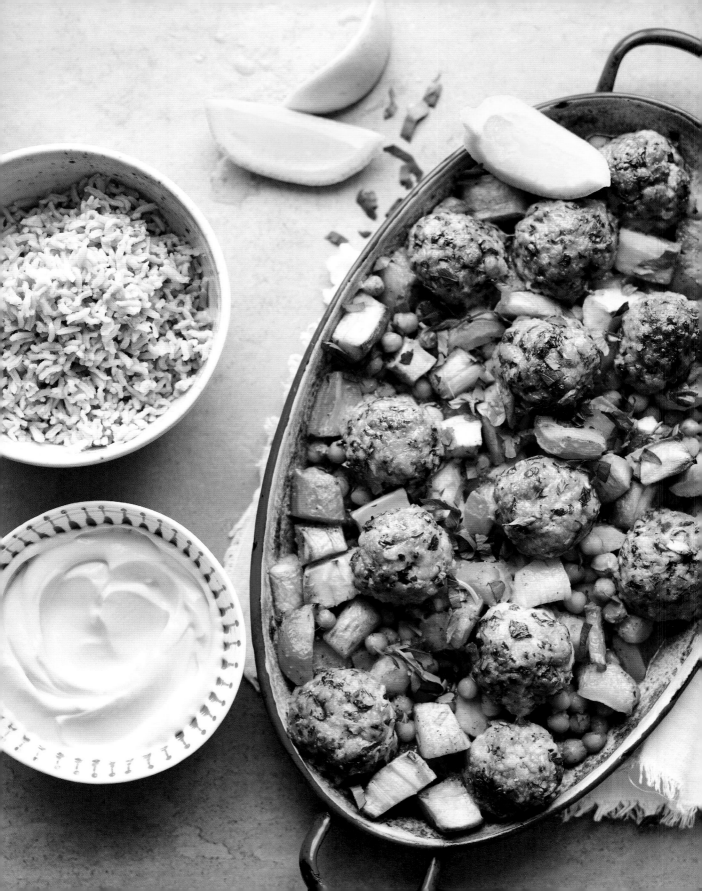

ONE-TRAY MEATBALLS WITH ROOT VEG & TOMATO BROTH

This is a great meal to serve in place of a Sunday roast or for a weekend lunch with friends. The meatballs soak up the wonderful sauce and become really juicy and tender. With lots of sweet roasted root veg and fibre-rich chickpeas, it's super-nutritious as well as tasty.

SERVES 4

350g carrots, cut into 3cm chunks

500g parsnips, cut into 3cm chunks

1 tbsp olive oil

1 onion, peeled

500g minced pork

1 tsp ground cumin

1 tsp dried oregano

½ tsp chilli flakes

handful of fresh flat-leaf parsley, roughly chopped

30g panko breadcrumbs

1 egg

500ml hot chicken stock

100g sun-dried tomato pesto

400g tin of chickpeas, drained and rinsed

salt

To Serve

4 tbsp 0%-fat Greek yoghurt

handful of fresh parsley, roughly chopped

400g cooked brown rice

1 lemon, cut into wedges

1 Preheat the oven to 200°C/180°C fan.

2 Toss the carrots and parsnips with the oil and a pinch of salt in a large roasting pan. Roast for 30 minutes until soft and starting to turn golden.

3 Coarsely grate the onion and squeeze over the sink to release some of the liquid. Add the grated onion to a medium bowl with the pork, cumin, oregano, chilli flakes, parsley, breadcrumbs, egg and ½ teaspoon of salt. Mix together until combined, then scoop heaped tablespoons of the mixture and roll into balls.

4 Stir together the hot stock and pesto in a jug and set aside.

5 Remove the roasting pan from the oven, add the chickpeas, pour the stock and pesto broth over the vegetables and arrange the meatballs on top. Bake for a further 15–20 minutes until the meatballs are cooked through.

6 Turn the oven to the grill setting and grill for 3–5 minutes until the tops of the meatballs are browned.

7 Remove from the oven, dollop on the yoghurt and scatter over the parsley. Serve with cooked rice, with lemon wedges for squeezing over.

FEEL GOOD FACT

Parsnips are a good source of fibre, and vitamins C and K.

MISO COD, SWEET POTATO & EDAMAME TRAYBAKE

This miso-coated cod is so beautiful, I could eat it every day. Edamame beans are actually soy beans, and they are a convenient way to add a plant-based source of protein to your meals, as well as being rich in many other essential micronutrients.

SERVES 4

800g sweet potatoes, peeled and cut into 3cm chunks

2 tbsp light olive oil

pinch of salt

2 tbsp white or brown miso paste

1 tbsp runny honey

1 tsp sesame oil

1½ tsp apple cider vinegar

½ tsp grated fresh ginger

150g frozen podded edamame beans

4 x 150g skinless cod fillets

2 tbsp sesame seeds

2 spring onions, thinly sliced

1 Preheat the oven to 200°C/180°C fan.

2 Toss the sweet potato chunks with the oil and salt on a large baking tray. Roast in the oven for 30 minutes, flipping them after 15 minutes.

3 Mix the miso, honey, sesame oil, vinegar and ginger in a bowl until smooth.

4 Remove the tray from the oven and add the frozen edamame and the cod fillets. Spread the miso mixture over the tops of each piece of cod and sprinkle everything with the sesame seeds. Return to the oven for 10–15 minutes until the cod is cooked through (it should be opaque in the centre).

5 Garnish with the thinly sliced spring onions and serve.

FEEL GOOD FACT

Cod is a low-fat source of protein and a good source of phosphorous, niacin and vitamin B12. It's particualrly good for maintaining our energy levels.

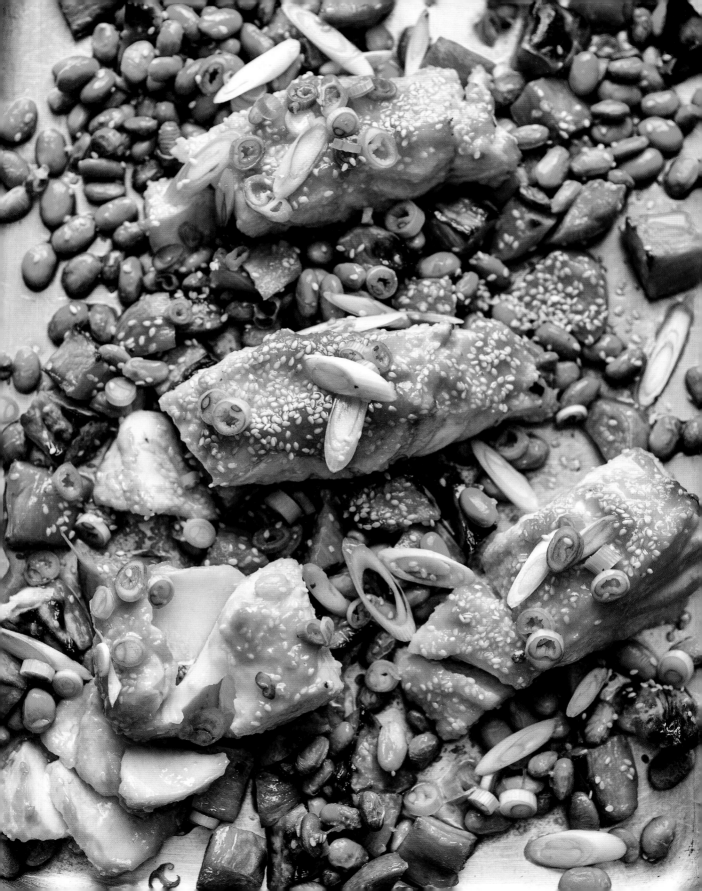

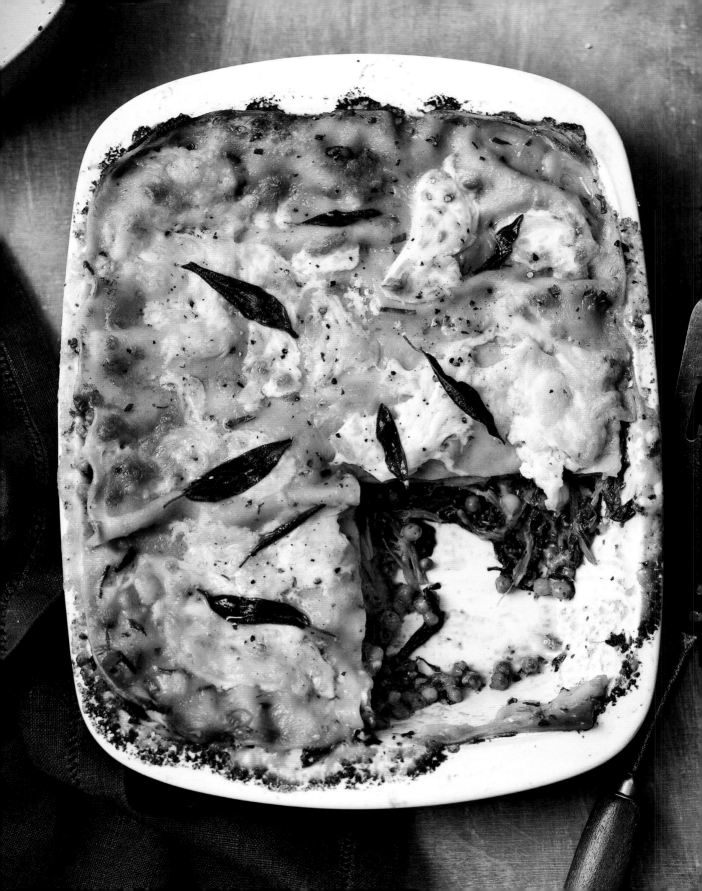

SPINACH, PEA & SAGE LASAGNE

I've made a few veggie lasagnes before, but this one is without a doubt my best creation yet. The sage and ricotta cheese give it such a luxurious and creamy taste. It can be prepared ahead of time and kept in the fridge to bake when you're ready, or frozen for up to a month and reheated in the oven (double the bake time if cooking from frozen).

SERVES 4–6

40g butter

1 tbsp roughly chopped fresh sage, plus 10–12 whole leaves, for garnish

40g plain or wholemeal flour

500ml vegetable stock (or chicken stock, if not vegetarian)

25g vegetarian hard cheese or Parmesan, finely grated

750g frozen whole-leaf spinach, defrosted

300g frozen peas, defrosted

250g ricotta cheese

150g green basil pesto

250g fresh lasagne sheets (or 250–300g dried lasagne sheets)

125-g ball of fresh mozzarella cheese

1 tsp light olive oil

freshly ground black pepper

1 Heat the butter in a medium saucepan over a medium heat until melted. Add the chopped sage leaves and cook for 1 minute to infuse the butter. Stir in the flour and cook for 1 minute to toast it, then gradually whisk in the stock until you get a smooth sauce. Stir in the cheese and set aside.

2 Place the defrosted spinach in a sieve set over a bowl or the sink. Squeeze as much liquid out of the spinach as possible, then tip into a medium bowl with the defrosted peas, ricotta and pesto. Stir together and set aside.

3 Preheat the oven to 200°C/180°C fan.

4 Spoon a third of the spinach mixture into a large baking dish and spread out to cover the base. Layer a quarter of the white sauce on top, then add a layer of lasagne sheets (you may need to tear/break the pasta sheets to get full coverage). Repeat the same layering process twice more, then pour the remaining white sauce over the pasta, tear over the mozzarella and sprinkle with the whole sage leaves. Drizzle with the olive oil and a grating of black pepper.

5 Bake for 35–45 minutes until the cheese is browned and the lasagne is bubbling.

BAKED RICOTTA-&-SPINACH-STUFFED PASTA SHELLS

Oh my word. Take a look at that photo. How delicious does that look? If you love pasta, this recipe is a dream for you. Ricotta and spinach are a proper match made in heaven. You are not going to be disappointed with this one, that's for sure.

SERVES 4

1 tbsp light olive oil

1 onion, diced

2 x 400g tins of chopped tomatoes

1 medium carrot, grated

1 tbsp balsamic vinegar

1 tsp dried oregano

300g giant pasta shells

350g frozen whole-leaf spinach, defrosted

250g ricotta cheese

1 tbsp green basil pesto

1 egg

20g vegetarian hard cheese or Parmesan, grated

salt and freshly ground black pepper

1 Heat the olive oil in a medium saucepan over a medium heat, add the onion and cook for about 10 minutes until softened and starting to turn golden. Add the chopped tomatoes, grated carrot, balsamic vinegar and dried oregano. Fill up one of the tomato tins with water and pour that into the pan, too. Bring to the boil over a high heat, then reduce to a simmer and cook for 30 minutes until the sauce has reduced a little. Remove from the heat.

2 If you like, give the sauce a few blitzes with a hand blender in the pan to break down any larger bits of tomato or carrot. Pour the sauce into a deep, 23 x 33cm (or similar size) baking dish and set aside.

3 Bring a large pan of well-salted water to the boil. Add the pasta and cook until al dente (usually about 1 minute less than the packet instructions state). Drain the pasta and rinse under cold water.

4 Preheat the oven to 200°C/180°C fan.

5 Place the defrosted spinach in a sieve and set it over the sink. Squeeze to remove as much moisture as possible from the spinach, then tip into a medium bowl. Add the ricotta, pesto, egg and a pinch of black pepper, and stir together until combined.

6 Fill each pasta shell with around a heaped teaspoonful of filling. Lay the filled shells on top of the sauce in the baking dish, overlapping them slightly (like shingled roof tiles), until you've used up all the filling. Sprinkle with the Parmesan and bake for 30 minutes until the sauce is thick and bubbling.

FEEL GOOD FACT

Tomatoes contain betacarotene (converted to vitamin A in body, and essential for eye and skin health, and improved immune system function), vitamin C (for maintaining skin health and the formation of collagen), and lycopene (an antioxidant that may be beneficial for cardiovascular health).

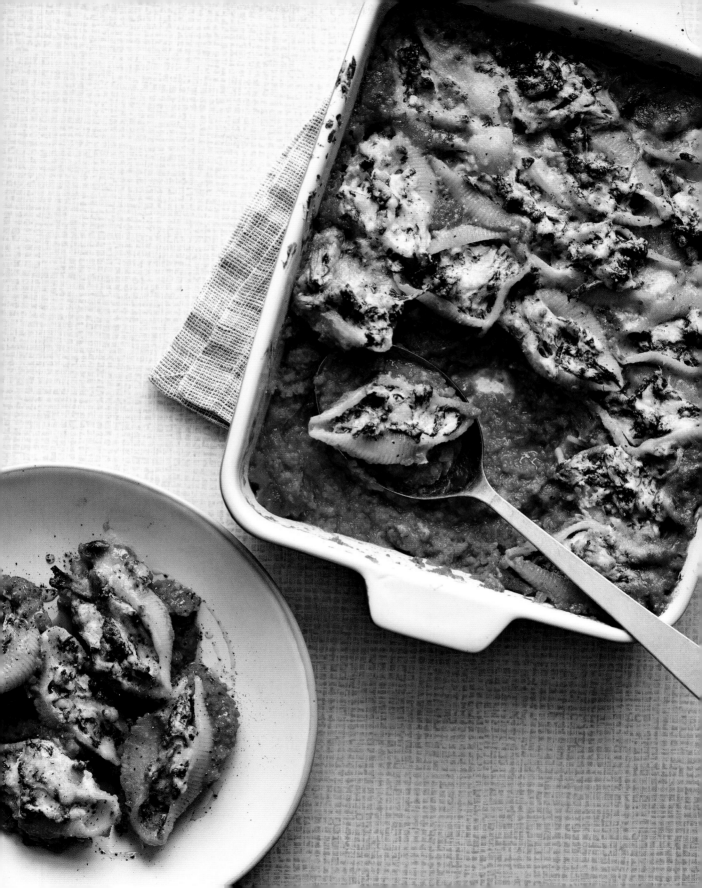

JOE'S WOW CHICKEN, CAULI, LEEK & BEAN PIE

Oh, guilty! Here he is... back with another filo-topped pie. Since my very first cookbook back in 2015, I have included a filo pie in every single book. I never thought I would be able to top the original Joe's Chicken Pie but I can honestly say this is the one. It takes the crown. It's so unbelievably creamy and rich. You are going to love this!

SERVES 4

1 head of cauliflower, leaves removed, cut into bite-sized florets

3 tbsp light olive oil, plus extra for drizzling

1 large leek, cleaned and cut into 2cm pieces

400g boneless, skinless chicken thighs, diced

3 tbsp plain or wholemeal flour

500ml hot chicken stock

200ml milk of choice

1 bay leaf

4 sprigs of fresh thyme, leaves picked

2 tbsp reduced-fat crème fraîche

400g tin of cannellini beans, drained and rinsed

6–8 sheets of filo pastry

salt and freshly ground black pepper

1 Preheat the oven to 200°C/180°C fan.

2 In a 2.5-litre pie dish or large roasting tray, toss the cauliflower with 1 tablespoon of the oil. Roast for 30 minutes until starting to turn golden brown.

3 Meanwhile, heat 1 tablespoon of the oil in a large frying pan over a medium-low heat. Add the leek and gently cook for 7–10 minutes until softened. Remove to a bowl and set aside.

4 Return the pan to the heat and add the remaining tablespoon of oil. Once hot, add the chicken pieces and cook until golden, turning as needed. Sprinkle the flour over the chicken in the pan and stir through, then gradually stir in the chicken stock, using a spoon to scrape up any golden crusty bits from the bottom of the pan. Once all the stock has been added, add the leeks back in along with the milk, bay leaf and thyme. Stir until the sauce thickens, then take off the heat and stir in the crème fraîche and cannellini beans. Remove and discard the bay leaf, then taste and season with salt and pepper.

5 Once the cauliflower is roasted, pour the contents of the pan into the pie dish/tray. Take a piece of filo pastry and scrunch it up in your hand. Place on top of the pie filling in the dish, then repeat with the remaining filo to cover the top of the pie. Drizzle with a little olive oil and bake for 25–30 minutes until the pastry is golden and crisp.

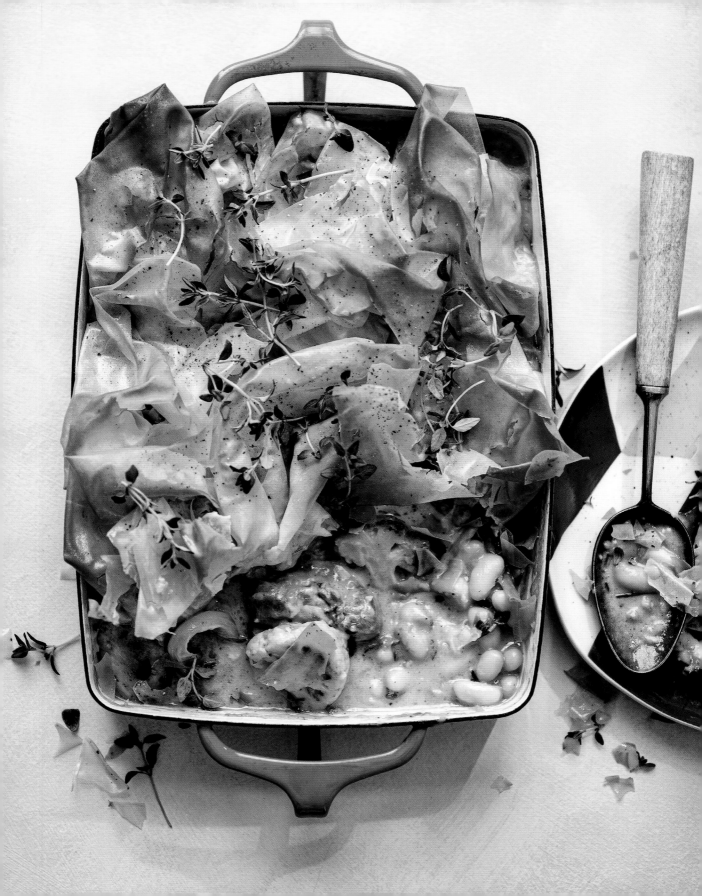

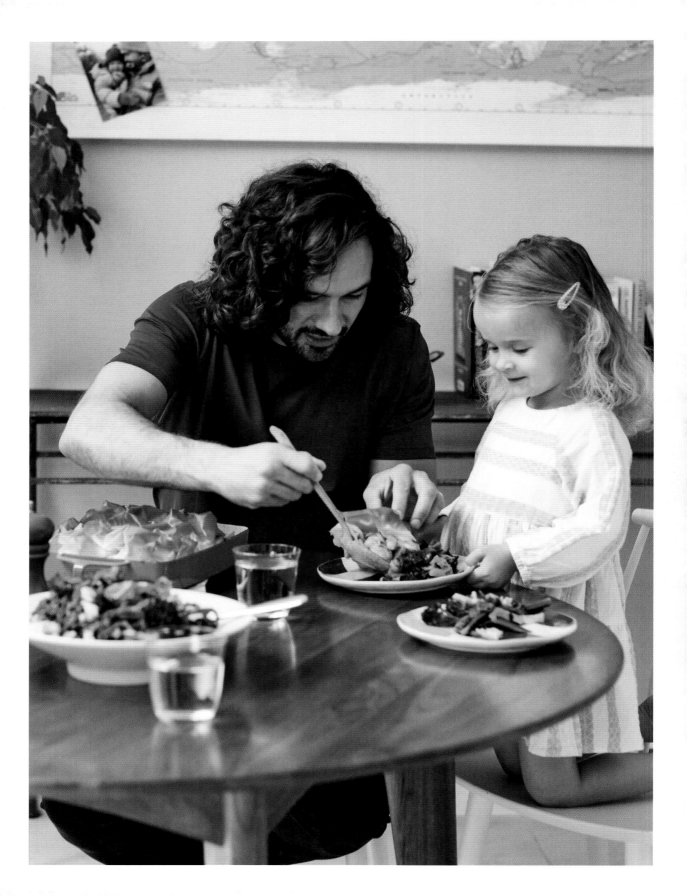

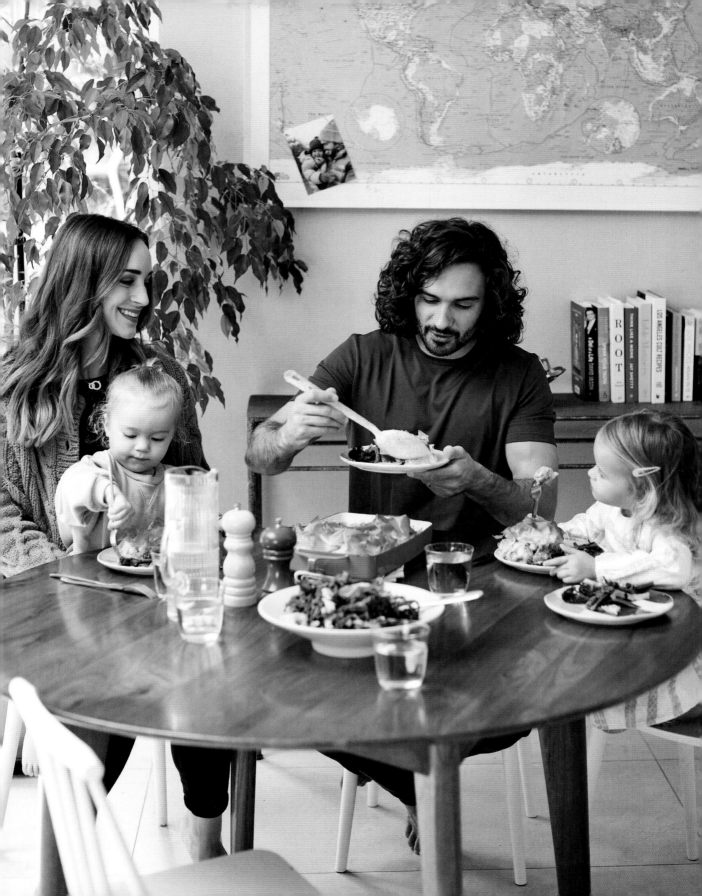

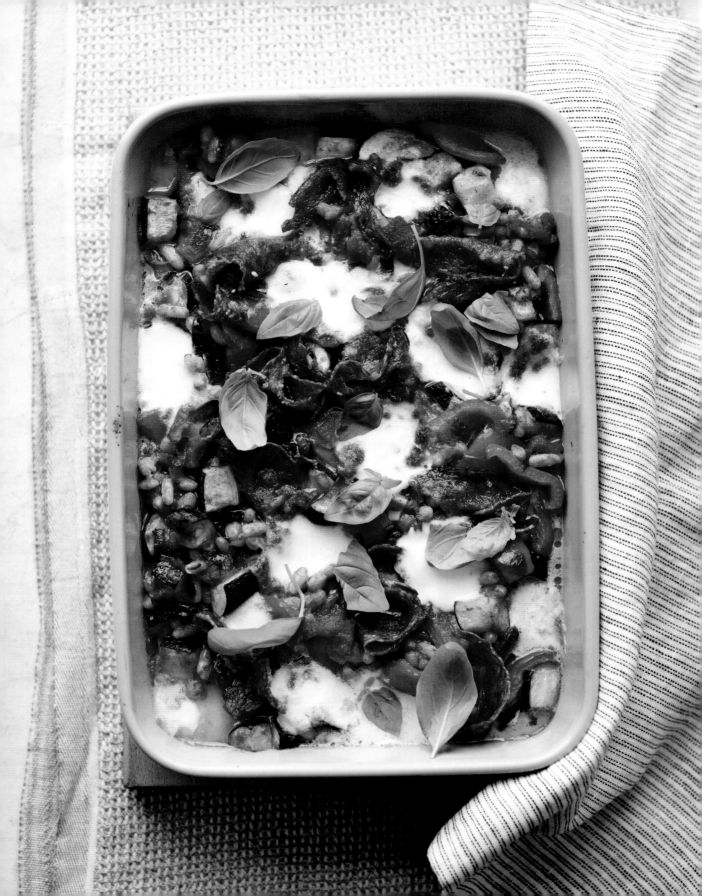

MEDITERRANEAN VEGETABLE, SALAMI & MOZZARELLA GRATIN

Imagine the flavours of a pizza in a creamy bean-based gratin. This delicious dish uses just a small amount of salami to bring some flavour and is rammed with healthy veg. You'll need a wide, deep, ovenproof frying pan; if you don't have an oven-safe one, use a medium ovenproof dish or a deep roasting tin.

SERVES 4

3 tbsp light olive oil

2 red onions, diced

2 red peppers, seeds removed, diced into 3cm chunks (or use 200g frozen sliced)

2 medium courgettes, diced into 3cm chunks

2 garlic cloves, crushed

400g tin of chopped tomatoes

400g tin of haricot beans, drained and rinsed

2 tsp dried oregano

1 tbsp balsamic vinegar

125g ball of fresh mozzarella

50g salami, thinly sliced (I really like a fennel salami)

a handful of fresh basil leaves, torn

salt

4 slices of crusty wholemeal bread, to serve

1 Heat a wide, deep, ovenproof frying pan over a medium-low heat and add 1 tablespoon of the oil. Once hot, add the onions, peppers and a pinch of salt. Cover with a lid and cook for 10–15 minutes, stirring occasionally, until the vegetables are starting to brown. Remove from the pan to a plate and set aside.

2 Return the pan to the heat. Add the remaining 2 tablespoons of oil along with the courgettes and another pinch of salt. Cook, uncovered, over a medium heat for about 10 minutes, stirring occasionally, until golden. Stir in the garlic, cook for 30 seconds, then add the chopped tomatoes, haricot beans, oregano, balsamic vinegar and the cooked onions and peppers. Cook for 5 minutes just to reduce the sauce slightly. Taste and adjust the seasoning with salt, if needed.

3 Meanwhile, preheat the grill to high.

4 If your pan isn't ovenproof, transfer the contents of the pan to an ovenproof dish now. Tear the mozzarella and scatter over the vegetables, then top with the slices of salami. Place under the grill to cook until the cheese has melted and is bubbling – watch it carefully as this will happen quite quickly. Once done, remove from the oven and sprinkle with the basil.

5 Serve the gratin with crusty bread for dipping.

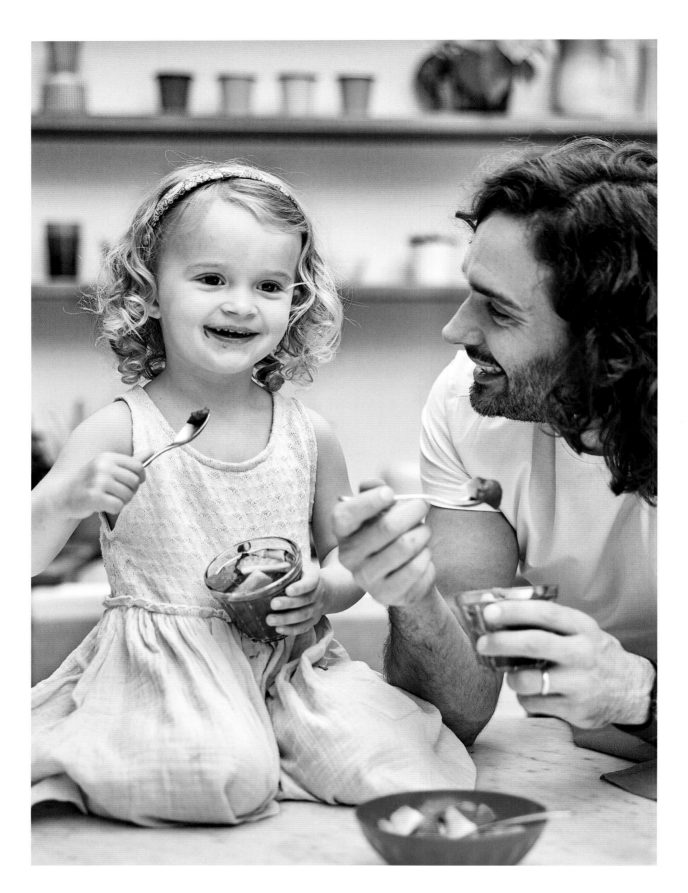

8

SWEET
TREATS

low-sugar desserts and energy bars
to give you a lift

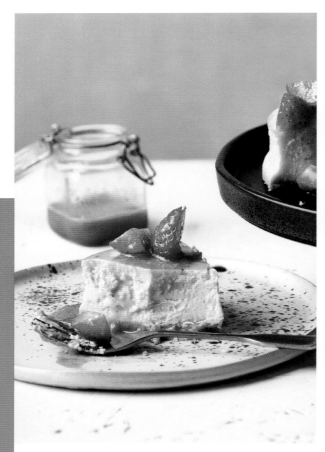
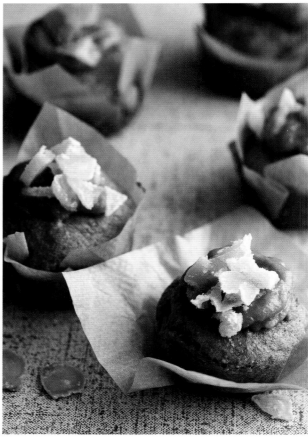

The ultimate feel good food experience just has to be sweet! I've definitely got a bit of a sweet tooth, so I'm excited for you to try these recipes, as they're ticking all my boxes for amazing flavour with less sugar and some healthy swaps too.

Whether you're looking for a small treat, such as an energy bar, a cookie or a cupcake, or whether you want a showstopper dessert to put on the table at a get-together, this chapter has got you covered.

Rosie and the kids love the Strawberry and Yoghurt Flapjacks on page 272. They're really good to pack in a box for a picnic or family walk, or to pop in a lunchbox for school or work. They're great for an energy boost and full of super-healthy ingredients – the ideal pick-me-up.

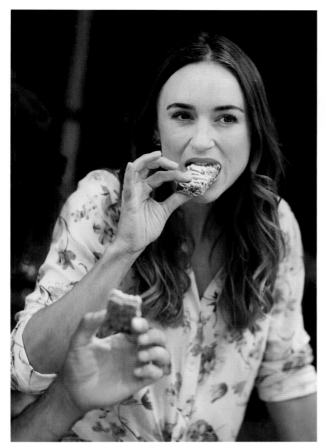
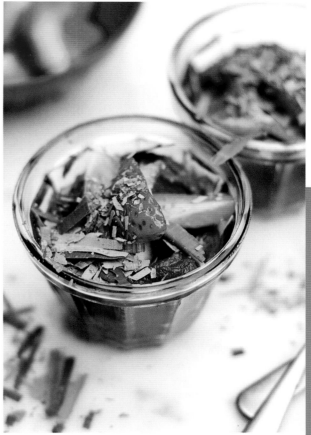

With Choc Chip Oat and Banana Cookies (page 278), a warming apple cobbler (page 294) and a really lovely Date, Walnut and Carrot Loaf Cake (page 288), there's plenty of those everyday treats that just make you feel warm and fuzzy.

There's a gorgeous and so-easy-I-can't-believe-it Mango, Coconut and Lime Sorbet recipe on page 282. And you'll be blown away by the Chocolate Sweet Potato Mousse on page 291. Indie and Marley pretty much inhale this and they'd never guess that the secret ingredient is healthy sweet potato if it wasn't for the fact that they love to help me make it. I love getting the kids involved in the kitchen and, with a bit of supervision, this one is great fun to do with them.

Finally, I'm OBSESSED with the Baked Ricotta and Strawberry Cheesecake on page 286. It's just awesome – I can't wait for you to try it.

STRAWBERRY & YOGHURT FLAPJACKS

These flapjacks are a really simple and healthy treat. Perfect for a school lunchbox or picnic. They really hit the spot for a sweet, yet filling, snack, providing fibre, healthy fats and protein. They're super-quick to make, too, only needing a very short bake to keep them moist and soft. Delicious!

MAKES 18

100g smooth almond or peanut butter

100g runny honey or golden syrup

2 tbsp coconut oil

50g ground almonds

200g jumbo oats

40g mixed seeds

pinch of salt

1 egg white

90g dried strawberries, roughly chopped

Yoghurt Coating

50g white chocolate

1½ tbsp coconut oil

2 tbsp natural yoghurt

1 tsp lemon juice

1 Preheat the oven to 200°C/180°C fan. Line a 23cm square cake tin with baking paper.

2 Melt the almond or peanut butter, honey or golden syrup and coconut oil together in a saucepan over a low heat until smooth. Remove from the heat and stir in the almonds, oats, seeds and salt. Finally, stir in the egg white and dried strawberries.

3 Tip the mixture into the prepared tin and press out into an even layer. Bake for 5 minutes until set around the edges but still soft.

4 Remove from the oven and cut into 18 bars with a sharp knife, then allow to cool completely.

5 To make the yoghurt coating, place the white chocolate and coconut oil in a small, heatproof bowl set over a small pan of simmering water. Stir occasionally until melted, then remove from the heat and allow to cool for 5 minutes. Mix in the yoghurt and lemon juice until smooth. Pour the mixture into a sandwich bag and snip off the corner to make a piping bag.

6 Drizzle the coating over the flapjack bars and leave to set. Store in an airtight container for up to 1 week.

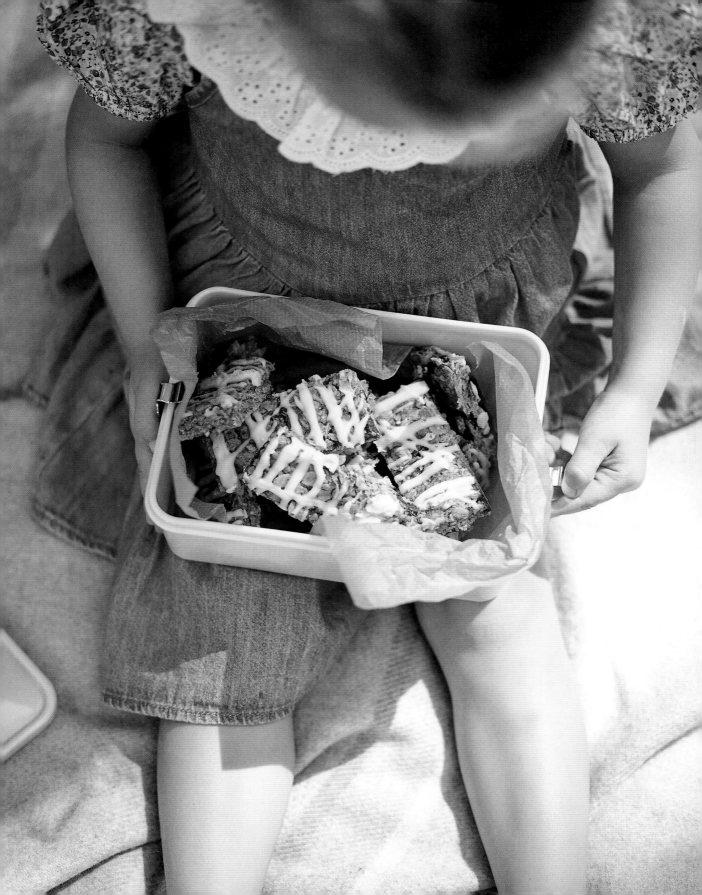

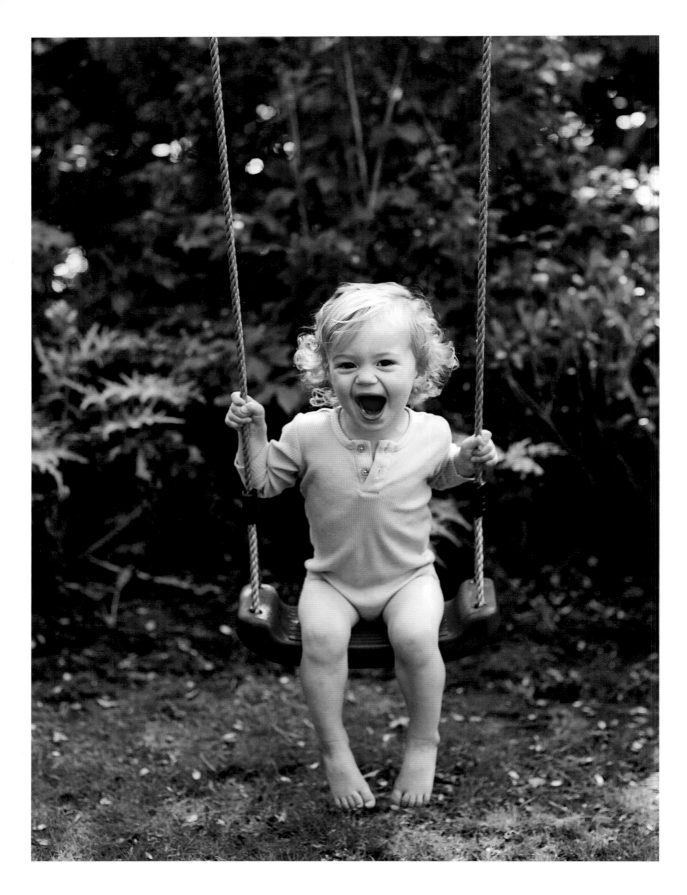

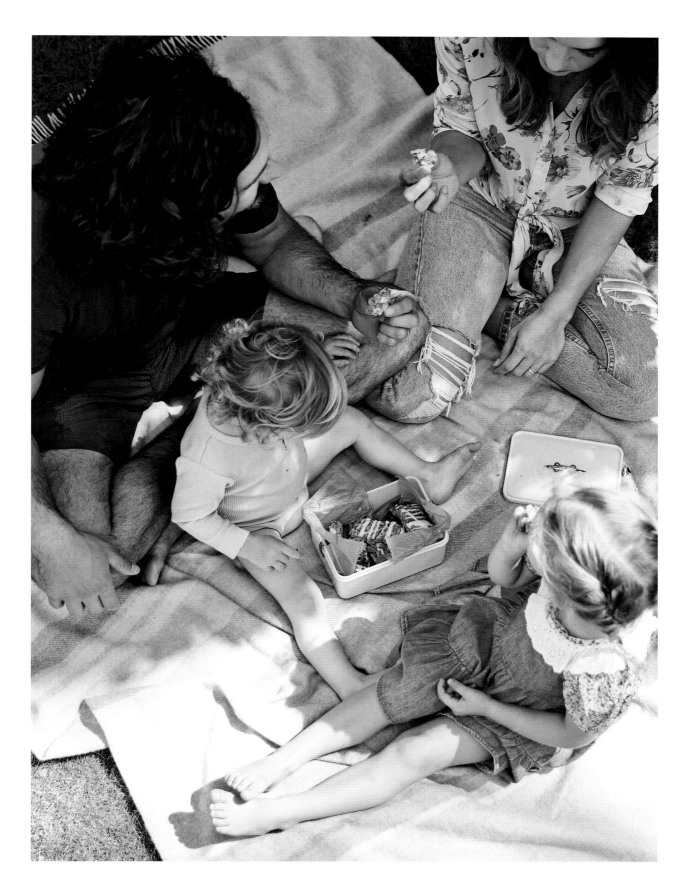

CHOCOLATE ORANGE POPCORN BITES

I really love making these with the kids. It's a messy business with lots of melted chocolate on noses and plenty of spoon licking going on, but it's so much fun. Beware – these bites are so incredibly moreish, you'll probably end up eating the whole batch in one sitting.

MAKES 12

45g salted popcorn

30g wholegrain puffed rice cereal (Rice Krispies)

80g runny honey

75g smooth almond butter

1 tbsp coconut oil

50g dark chocolate (70% cocoa solids), chopped

finely grated zest of 1 orange

2 tbsp chopped pistachios, to decorate (optional)

1 Line a 12-cup muffin tin with paper cases.

2 Place the popcorn and puffed rice into a large bowl.

3 Heat the honey in a small saucepan over a high heat until it starts to bubble. Reduce the heat to low and let it bubble away for 1–2 minutes until slightly darkened and fragrant. Stir in the almond butter, coconut oil and chocolate until melted, then remove from the heat.

4 Set ½ teaspoon of the orange zest aside for garnish and stir the rest into the melted chocolate mixture.

5 Pour the chocolate mixture over the popcorn and puffed rice. Use two spoons to toss the mixture together until everything is coated.

6 Divide the mixture between the lined muffin cups. Sprinkle with the remaining orange zest and the pistachios, if using. Leave to set at room temperature before eating. They will keep for about 2–3 days in an airtight container.

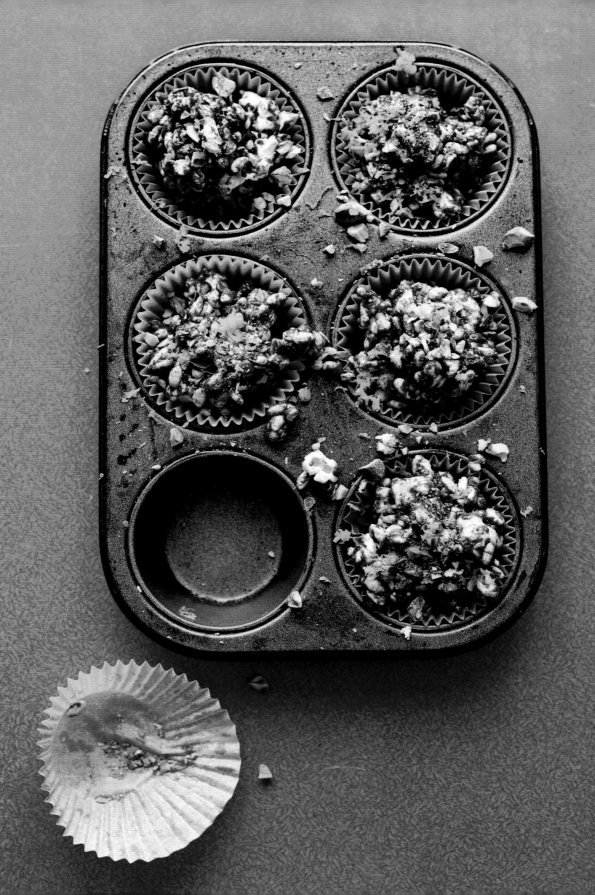

CHOCOLATE CHIP, OAT & BANANA COOKIES

Hello... did someone say cookies? I've got such a sweet tooth, so these always go down a storm in my house. They contain peanut butter and dark chocolate, so you can imagine how good they taste. Time to get baking!

MAKES 12–14

200g ripe, peeled bananas

120g smooth peanut butter

2 tbsp runny honey

1 tsp baking powder

135g porridge oats

100g dark chocolate (70% cocoa solids)

1 Preheat the oven to 200°C/180°C fan and line a baking tray with baking paper.

2 Mash the peeled bananas with the back of a fork on a plate until smooth.

3 Mix the peanut butter and honey in a medium bowl, then stir in the mashed banana, followed by the baking powder and oats. Chop the chocolate into small chunks and mix into the dough.

4 Scoop tablespoonfuls of dough onto the baking tray, spacing them about 3cm apart. Bake for 7–10 minutes until the edges are golden and set but the cookies are still soft.

5 Transfer the cookies to a wire rack to cool. Store in an airtight container for up to 4 days.

JOE'S TIPS

- Instead of the peanut butter, you can use your favourite nut butter.
- If you have a nut allergy, use tahini in place of the peanut butter.
- Add 1 tbsp unsweetened cocoa powder to the dough to make double chocolate cookies.
- Swap the chocolate for the same weight of raisins and add ½ tsp ground cinnamon for oat and raisin cookies.

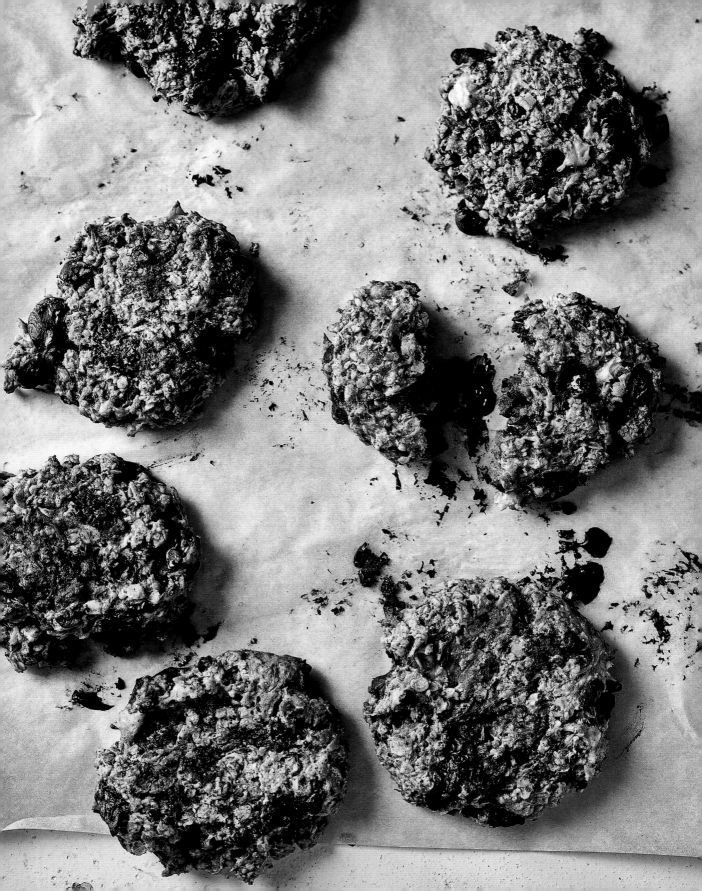

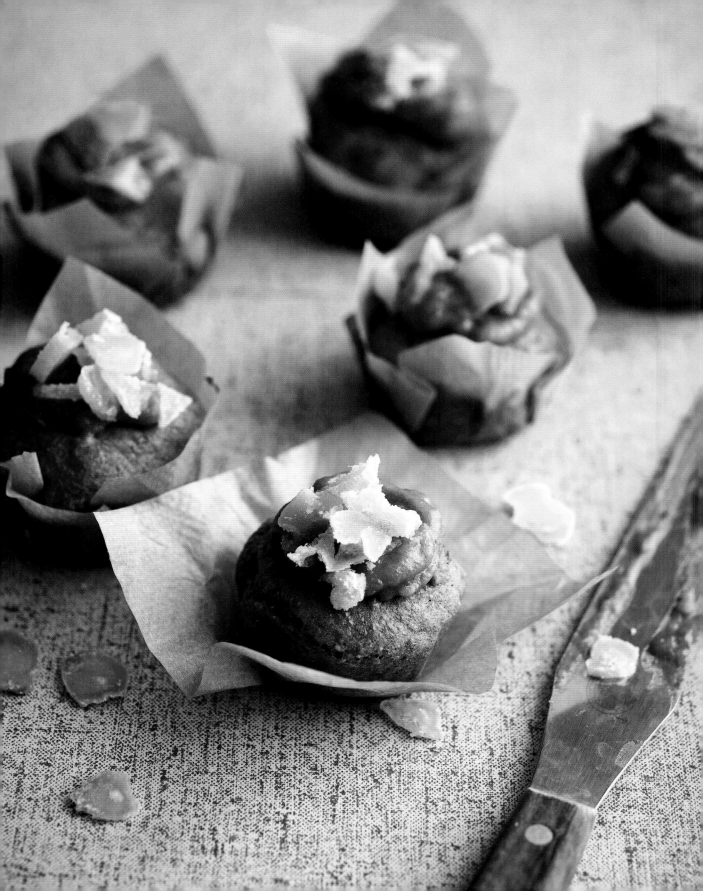

GINGERBREAD CUPCAKES WITH DATE CARAMEL

Who doesn't like gingerbread!? I've made these a few times for the kids at parties and they always go down very well. The date topping is genius, too. When soaked in hot water, the dates soften and can be blended into a purée, which has a smooth, sticky texture and a caramel-like flavour.

MAKES 6

90g wholemeal plain flour

30g soft dark brown sugar or coconut sugar

25g ground almonds

½ tsp baking powder

¼ tsp bicarbonate of soda

½ tsp ground cinnamon

1 tsp ground ginger

⅛ tsp ground clove

⅛ tsp ground nutmeg

pinch of salt

90g 0%-fat Greek yoghurt

45ml water

1 egg

1½ tbsp melted coconut oil

2 tbsp crystallised ginger chunks, to decorate

Date Caramel

100g pitted dates

60ml milk or non-dairy milk

1 tsp vanilla extract

good pinch of salt

1 Preheat the oven to 200°C/180°C fan and line a standard muffin tin with 6 muffin cases.

2 Mix together the flour, sugar, ground almonds, baking powder, bicarbonate of soda, spices and salt in a medium bowl.

3 In a separate bowl or jug, combine the yoghurt, water, egg and coconut oil.

4 Pour the wet mixture into the dry mixture and stir together until just combined. Divide the mixture between the prepared muffin cases.

5 Bake for 20–25 minutes until lightly browned on top and a toothpick inserted into the centre of a cupcake comes out clean. Set aside to cool.

6 Meanwhile, make the caramel. Place the dates into a small jug and cover with boiling water. Set aside for 15 minutes to soak.

7 Drain the dates and return to the jug, then add the milk, vanilla and salt. Blend until smooth with a hand blender, or in a food processor or free-standing blender.

8 Once you're ready to serve the cupcakes, frost them with the date caramel and sprinkle on some of the crystallised ginger chunks for decoration.

MANGO, COCONUT & LIME SORBET

This super-easy, creamy sorbet is delicious and is made with dairy-free coconut yoghurt, so it's great for anyone who can't handle dairy. When frozen and puréed, mango gets a smooth, silky texture, meaning you don't need an ice-cream machine. This tastes amazing on its own or served with some fresh berries.

SERVES 4

400g tin of mango slices in juice or syrup or 245g ripe, peeled mango flesh

150g dairy-free coconut yoghurt or low-fat Greek yoghurt if not vegan

juice of 1 lime

1 Drain the tinned mango, if using, reserving the juice/syrup from the tin (see Tips). Chop the mango flesh into bite-sized chunks and freeze in a freezer-safe container for 3 hours or until solid.

2 Tip the frozen mango chunks into the bowl of a food processor along with the yoghurt and half of the lime juice. Blitz until smooth and creamy.

3 Taste and add more lime juice, if needed.

4 Either serve immediately as a soft-serve sorbet or transfer to a lidded freezer-safe container and freeze for 1–2 hours until firm but still scoopable.

JOE'S TIPS

- You can buy already frozen mango chunks, however these can vary wildly in sweetness. If you do use them, make sure you taste the mixture after blitzing and adjust the sweetness to taste with some maple syrup or runny honey, as needed.
- If you use tinned mango, use the reserved syrup/juice for drizzling over fresh fruit and yoghurt for dessert. Or, for the adults, use it in a cocktail for a fruity flavour.

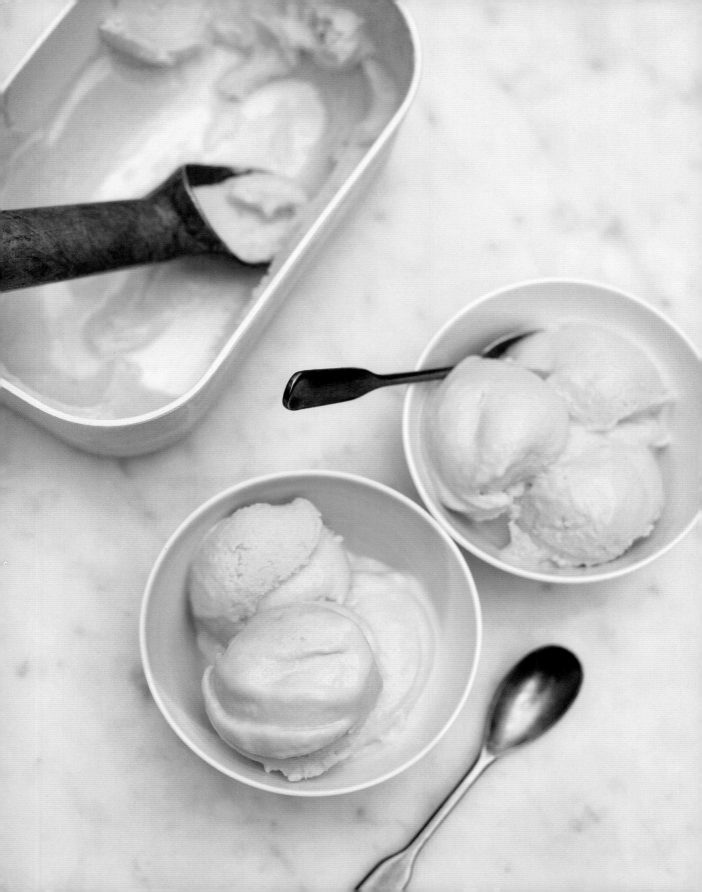

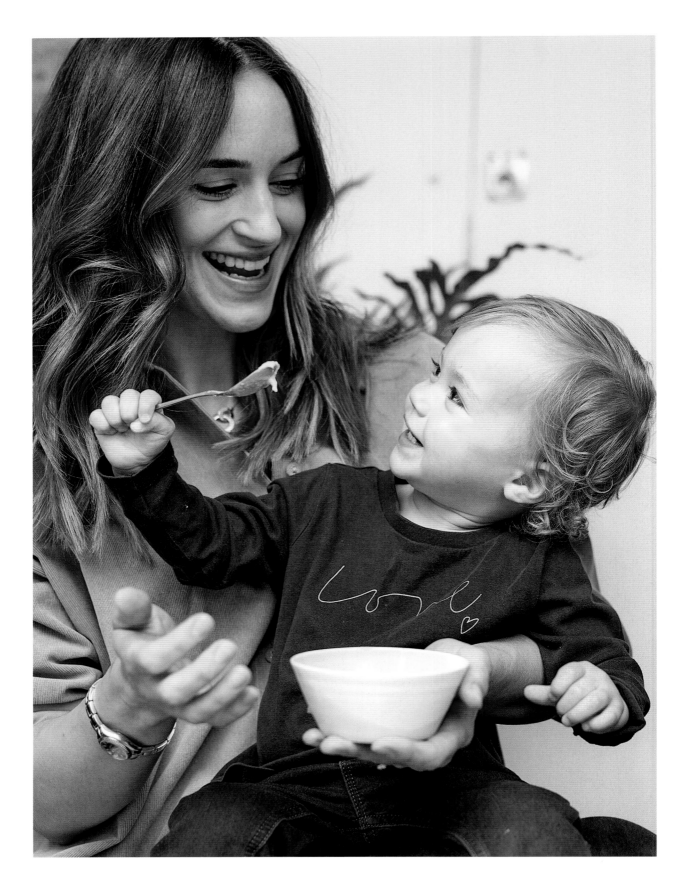

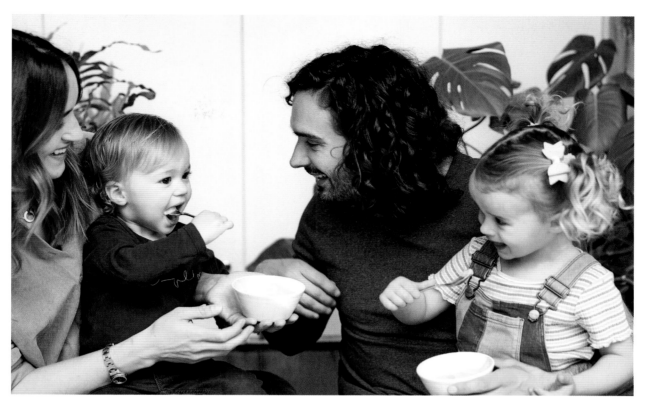
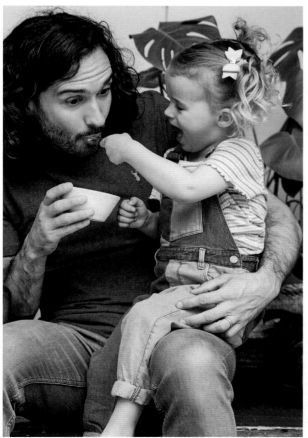
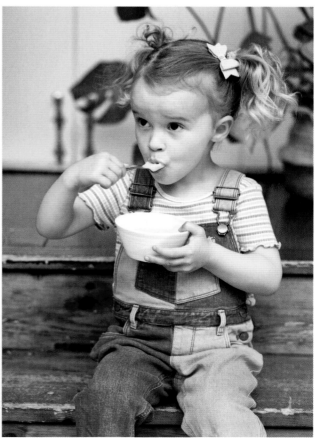

BAKED RICOTTA & STRAWBERRY CHEESECAKE

Cheesecake? Oh, yes please! This is a real showstopper, so if you have friends coming over or a party coming up, pull this recipe out. It's tangy, refreshing and creamy and I'll bet everyone loves it.

SERVES 8–10

Base

35g unsalted butter, melted
75g ground almonds
25g plain white flour
pinch of salt
1½ tsp caster sugar

Cheesecake Filling

250g ricotta cheese
340g light cream cheese
100g caster sugar
2 tbsp cornflour
3 large eggs
finely grated zest and juice of 1 lemon
1 tsp vanilla extract

Strawberry Topping

400g strawberries, hulled
2 tsp runny honey
1 tbsp lemon juice

1 Preheat the oven to 200°C/180°C fan. Use some of the melted butter to grease the sides of an 18cm springform cake tin.

2 Mix all of the base ingredients together in a medium bowl. Tip into the cake tin and press down into an even layer. Bake for 6–8 minutes until golden, then remove from the oven and set aside.

3 Turn the oven down to 160°C/140°C fan.

4 Sandwich the ricotta cheese between 4 layers of kitchen paper, patting it down to form a flat circle (this removes excess moisture from the cheese). Uncover and tip into a large bowl, then add the cream cheese and use a whisk to stir until smooth. Mix in the sugar and cornflour followed by the eggs, lemon zest and juice, and vanilla.

5 Pour the cheesecake filling over the baked crust and place the tin onto a baking tray. Bake for 50–60 minutes until the edges are set and the middle has a slight wobble. Carefully slide a knife around the outer edge of the baked cheesecake, then set aside to cool completely.

6 Meanwhile, make the strawberry topping. Tip 100g of the strawberries into a food processor with the honey and blitz until you have a smooth purée. Cut the remaining strawberries into quarters and place in a medium bowl. Add the strawberry purée and stir to coat.

7 Cut the cooled cheesecake into wedges and serve with the strawberry topping spooned over.

FEEL GOOD FACT

Ricotta is lower in salt than cream cheese, so swapping out some of the cream cheese for ricotta in a cheesecake can make it healthier (excess salt in the diet leads to high blood pressure).

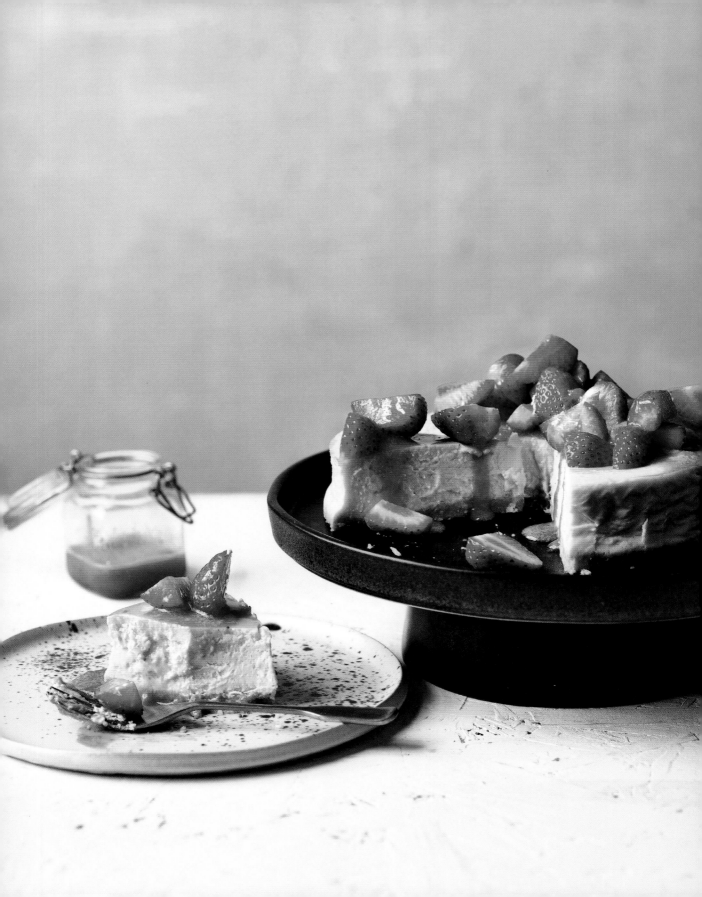

DATE, WALNUT & CARROT LOAF CAKE

Oh my word, I love this recipe! I make it every few weeks and it's always gone by the end of the day. The kids and Rosie help me eat it, of course! This is certainly something you'll want to make again and again.

SERVES 10–12

200g pitted dates, roughly chopped

2 tbsp coconut oil

125ml boiling water

1 tsp vanilla extract

½ tsp salt

80g runny honey

3 eggs

100g carrots, coarsely grated

180g plain wholemeal flour

100g walnuts, chopped

1 tsp bicarbonate of soda

¼ tsp salt

1 Preheat the oven to 200°C/180°C fan and line a 900g/2lb loaf tin with baking paper.

2 Add the chopped dates to a bowl along with the coconut oil. Pour over the boiling water and set aside for 10 minutes to soak (but do not drain).

3 Add the vanilla, salt, honey and eggs to the soaked dates, stirring together until combined.

4 In a separate bowl, combine the grated carrots, flour, walnuts, bicarbonate of soda and salt. Pour the wet mixture into the dry mixture and stir together until just combined.

5 Pour the batter into the loaf tin and bake for 50–60 minutes, covering the tin with foil for the last 30 minutes to prevent the cake browning too much.

6 Cool in the tin for 10 minutes, then tip out onto a wire rack and leave to cool completely before slicing.

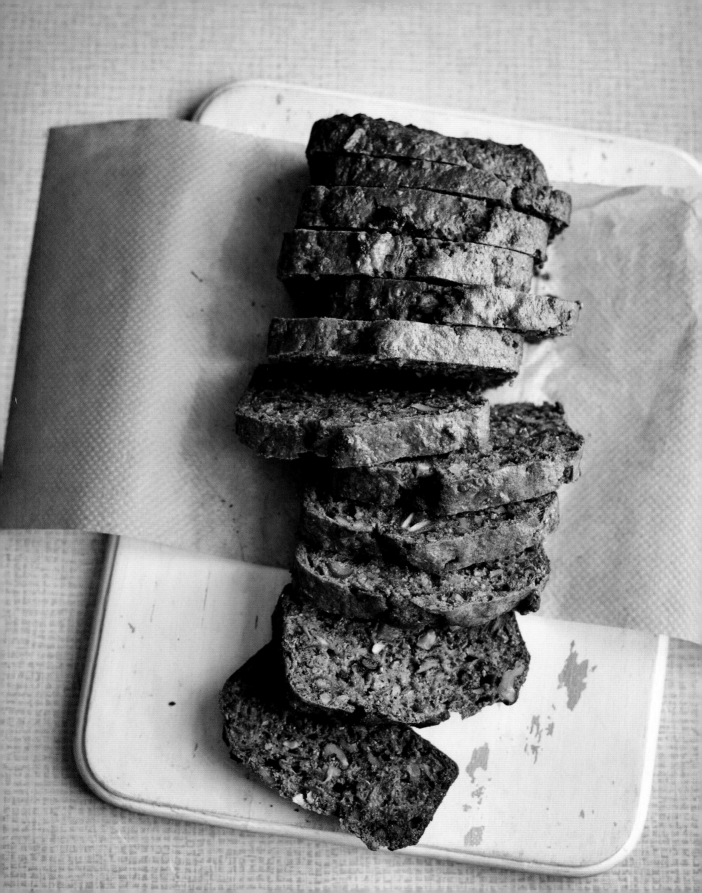

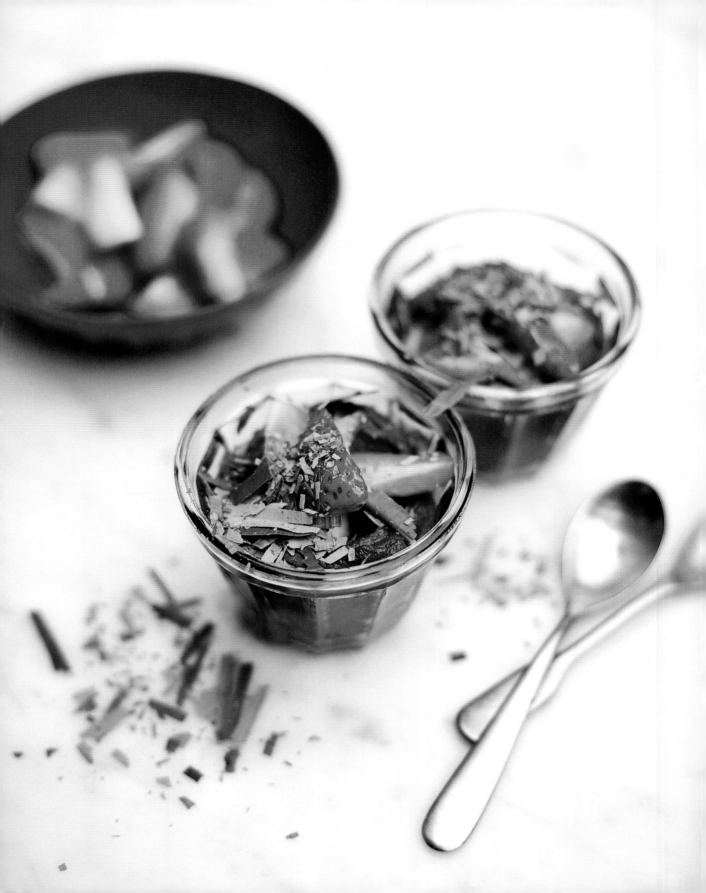

CHOCOLATE SWEET POTATO MOUSSE

This is a fantastic recipe to make with children, who might find it hard to believe that the secret to this dark, rich, chocolatey mousse is sweet potato. It might seem strange, but honestly the sweetness and texture is unreal. If you like sweet treats, this one will be right up your street.

SERVES 4

450–500g (2 medium) sweet potatoes
150g dark chocolate (70% cocoa solids)
1 tsp vanilla extract
pinch of salt

To Serve

200g strawberries, sliced
1 tsp sugar, honey or maple syrup

1 Preheat the oven to 170°C/150°C fan.

2 Prick the sweet potatoes all over with a fork and place on a baking tray. Roast for 1–1½ hours until super-soft. Leave to cool a little.

3 Once cool enough to handle but still hot, cut the sweet potatoes in half and scoop the flesh into the bowl of a food processor.

4 Use a vegetable peeler to shave some of chocolate into curls and set aside for decoration. Break the remaining chocolate into small chunks and add to the bowl of the food processor with the vanilla and salt. Blitz until the chocolate has melted and combined with the warm sweet potato into a smooth purée.

5 Divide the mousse between 4 small glasses or ramekins and chill for at least 30 minutes (or for up to 2 days).

6 Just before you're about to serve, combine the sliced strawberries and sugar (or honey/maple syrup) in a medium bowl and stir. Set aside for 15 minutes so the strawberries can become juicy.

7 Top each glass of mousse with some of the strawberries and sprinkle with the chocolate curls.

JOE'S TIP

The mousse mixture makes a great stand-in for chocolate buttercream on cakes. You can loosen it with a bit of milk, if needed.

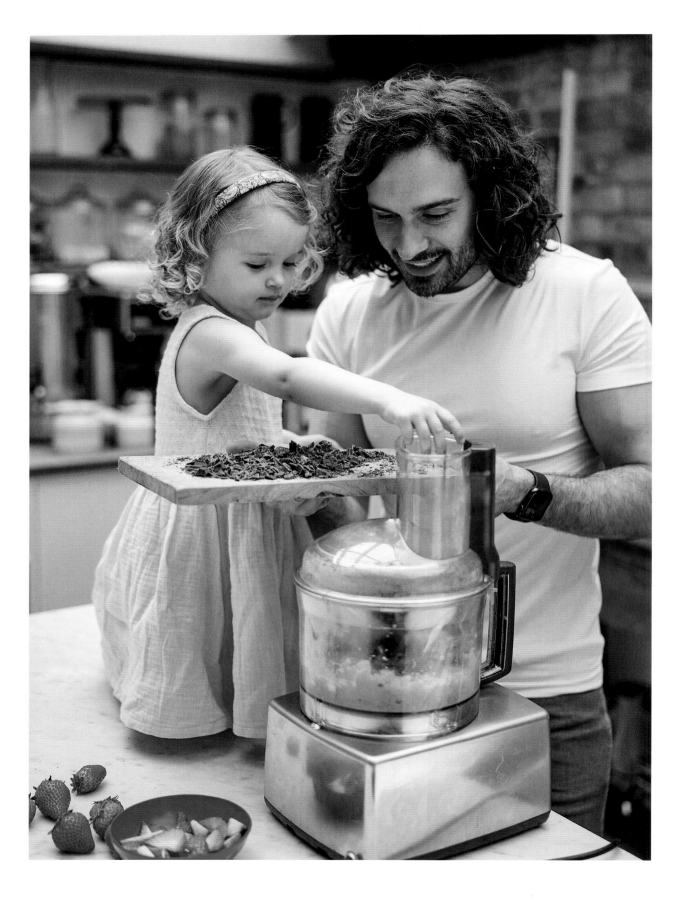

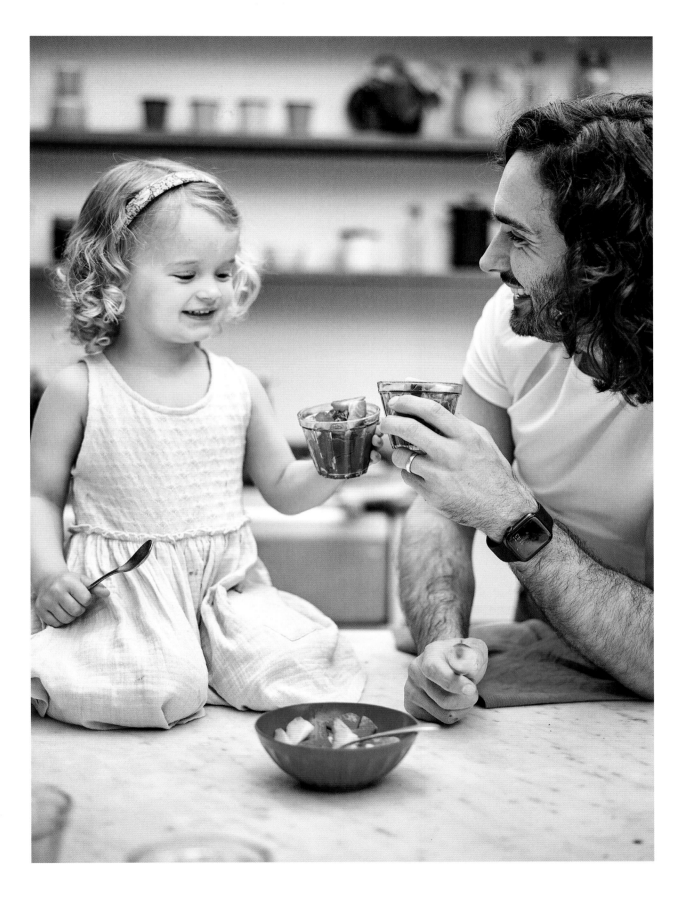

APPLE, GINGER & DATE COBBLER

WOW. Just look at that photo. Is that a bit of you? This comforting, sweet pudding is totally delicious. Great for one of those cold winter days where you want something to warm you up and put a big smile on your face. Cobbler me!

SERVES 6–8

Filling

75g pitted dates

100ml water

6 eating apples

1 tbsp cornflour

juice of ½ lemon

4 chunks of stem ginger in syrup, roughly chopped

Topping

70g plain white flour

3 tbsp coconut sugar

1 tsp baking powder

½ tsp ground cinnamon

¼ tsp salt

50g unsalted butter

60g jumbo oats

70g 0%-fat Greek yoghurt, plus extra to serve (optional)

1 egg

1 Preheat the oven to 200°C/180°C fan.

2 Place the dates and water in a small saucepan and cover with a lid. Simmer for 10–15 minutes until the dates are soft enough to be mashed with the back of a fork. Mash the dates into a rough paste, then remove from the heat and set aside.

3 Peel the apples, remove the cores and cut into 2cm chunks. Tumble the apple chunks into a 21 x 26cm baking dish along with the mashed dates, cornflour, lemon juice and stem ginger pieces. Toss everything together with your hands.

4 Cover the dish with foil and bake for 20 minutes until the apples are softened.

5 For the topping, combine the flour, coconut sugar, baking powder, cinnamon and salt in a medium bowl. Add the butter and rub together with your fingertips until sandy. Stir in the oats, then add the yoghurt and egg and mix until just combined into a thick batter.

6 Uncover the apples and dot the batter all over the top, spreading it out a bit with the back of a spoon so it's not too thick. Return to the oven for 25–30 minutes, until the topping is cooked through and the apples are soft.

7 Eat warm with yoghurt, if desired.

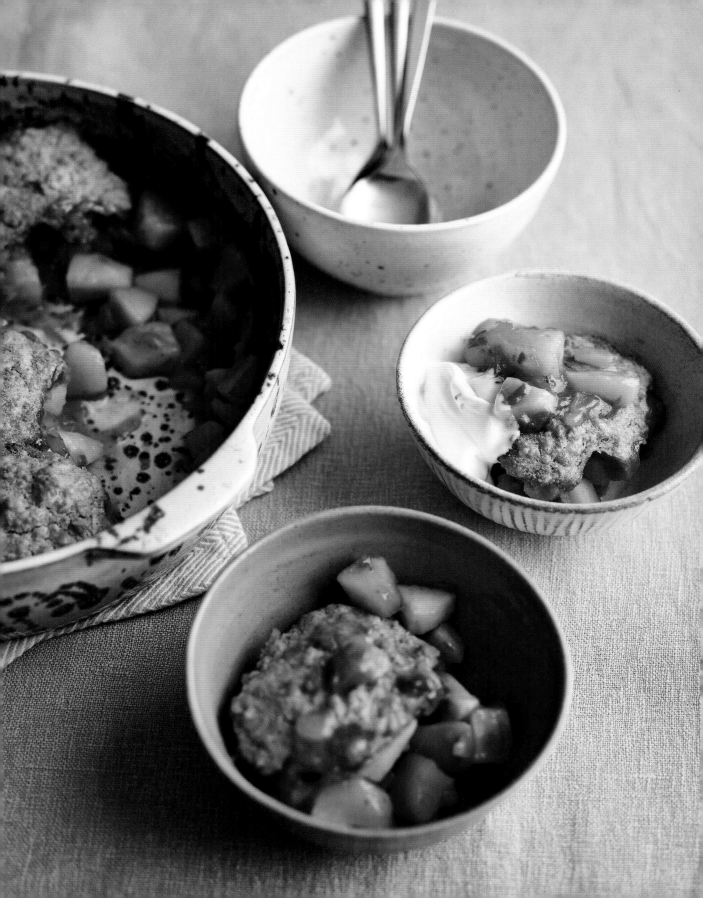

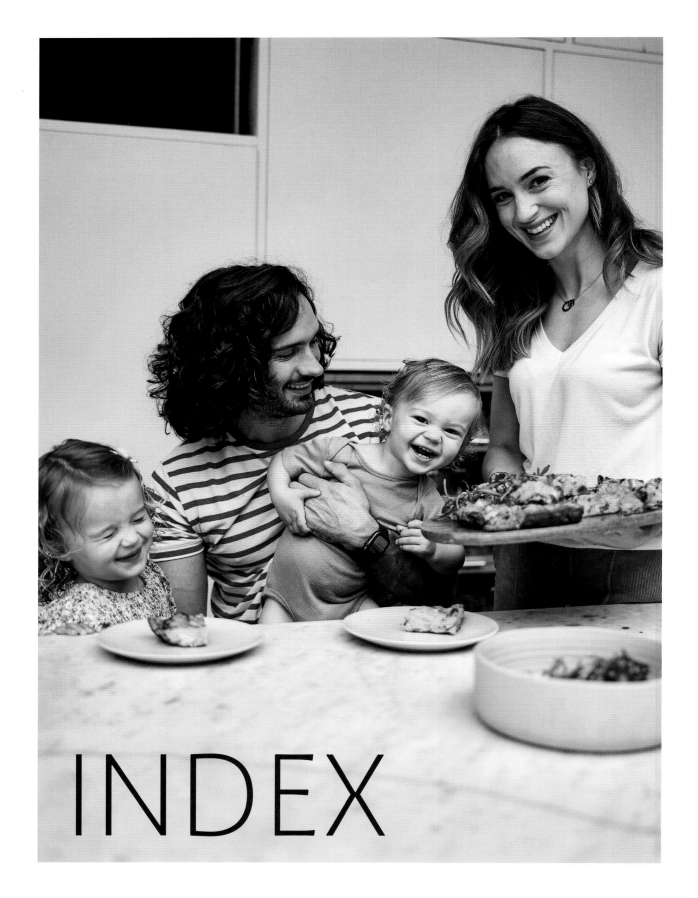

INDEX

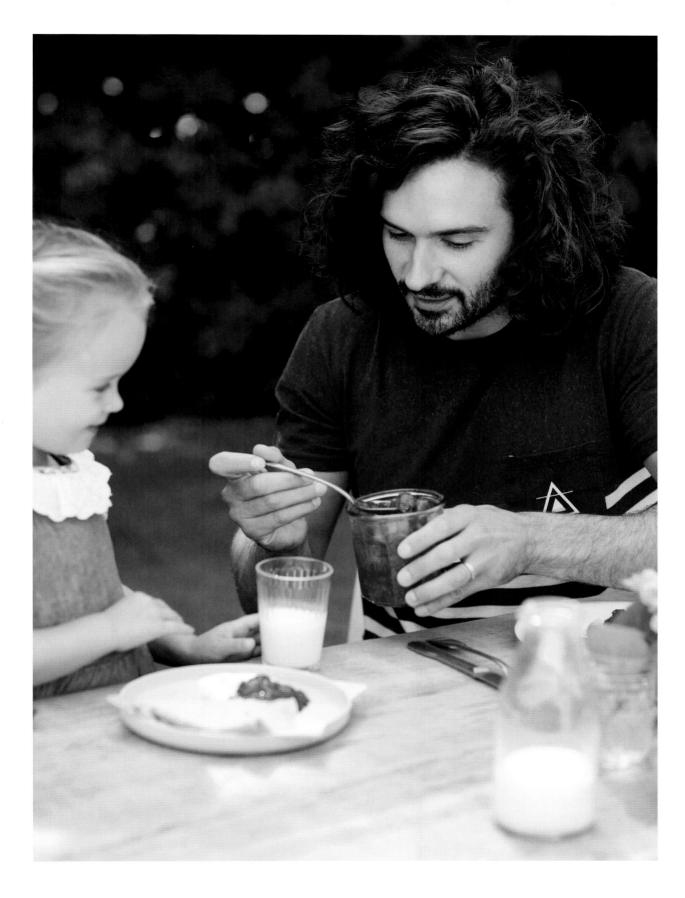

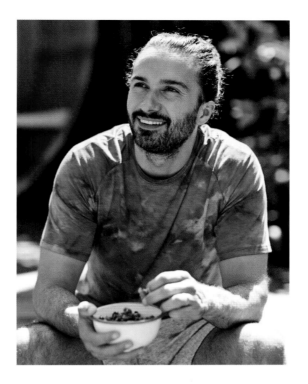

ACKNOWLEDGEMENTS

I'm so unbelievably proud of this book. I love everything about it, from the cover to the page design, food styling and images. A great book only comes together with a great team, so I want to say thank you to everyone involved in its creation.

To my wonder agent, Bev James, thank you for helping me bring this book to life – one of many books together. Thank you to Lisa Milton for bringing me to HarperCollins and giving me a wonderful opportunity to create more books. You're a pleasure to work with and I can't wait to see what we can achieve together in the future. Thank you to Emily and Kate for your amazing support on this book, too. It's really been such a great team effort. Thank you to Izy for the recipe advice and to Louise for the gorgeous page design. Finally, many thanks to Dan, Joss, Tamara, Kitty, Faye and Charlie, for creating the most stunning recipe images – I think everyone will love your photos and want to eat everything, just as I do.

Thank you!

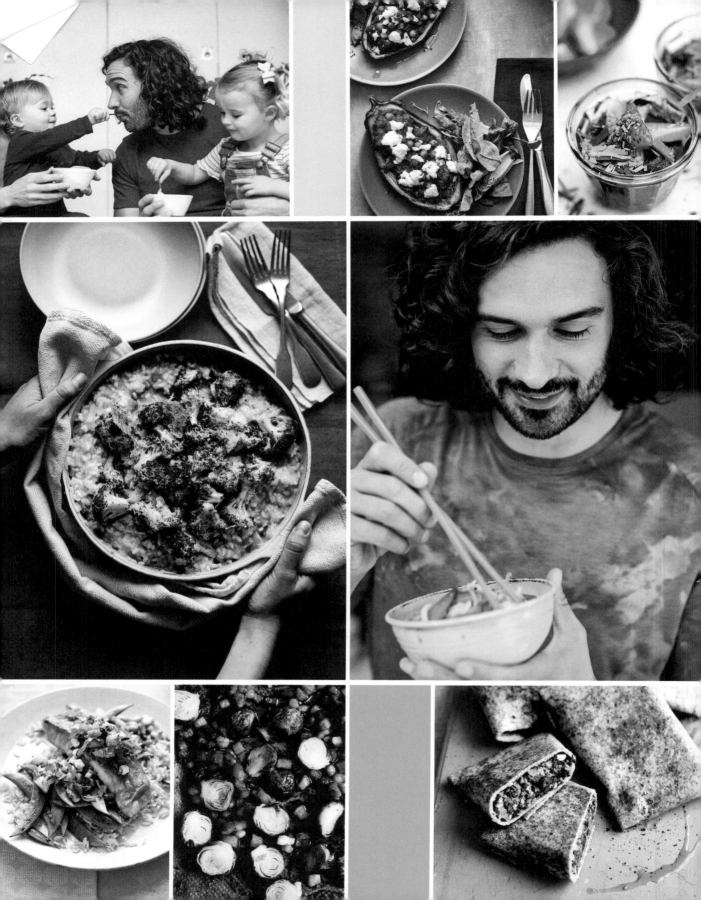